Pilates on the BOSU®

Fundamentals

by Miriane Taylor

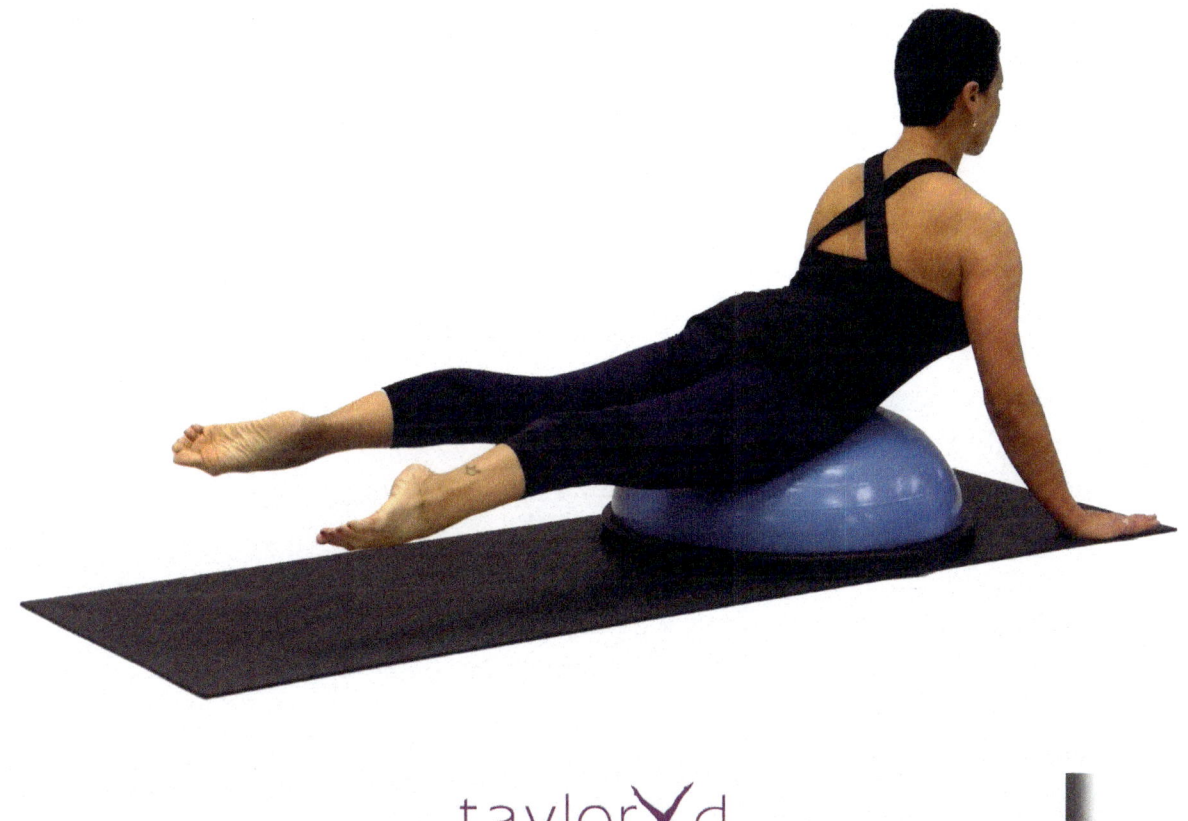

taylor'd PILATES   www.taylor-dpilates.com

Copyright © 2021 by Taylor'd Pilates

All information contained in this document is the property of Taylor'd Pilates. Duplication of any or all information is restricted without consent from Taylor'd Pilates or one of its representatives.

General Disclaimer:
This book has been written and published strictly for informational purposes, and in no way should be used as a substitute for consultation with health care professionals. You should not consider educational material herein to be the practice of medicine or to replace consultation with a physician or other medical practitioner. The author and publisher are providing you with information in this work so that you can have the knowledge and can choose, at your own risk, to act on that knowledge. The author and publisher also urge all readers to be aware of their health status and to consult health care professionals before beginning any health program.

TABLE OF CONTENTS

INTRODUCTIONS

TABLE OF CONTENTS	2
ACKNOWLEDGMENTS	4
FORWARD BY COLLEEN CRAIG	5
MY BOSU® JOURNEY	7
PARTS OF THE BOSU®	9
WHAT IS A BOSU®?	10
WHY PILATES ON THE BOSU®	10
THE 6 ORIGINAL PRINCIPLES OF PILATES TRAINING	11
THE 6 TAYLOR'D PILATES PRINCIPLES	11
PRACTICING SAFE BOSU®	15
ADVANTAGES OF USING THE BOSU®	16
PILATES APPROACH TO USING THE BOSU® BENEFITS	16
LAYOUT OF THE EXERCISES	16
DESCRIPTION OF THE FUNDAMENTAL LEVEL	17

EXERCISES

(1) SPINAL MOBILIZATION	18
(2) HIP RELEASE	21
(3) ARCH AND CURL SPINE	23
(4) CIRCLE UPPER BODY	25
(5) TIP UPPER BODY SIDE TO SIDE	28
(6) SCAPULAE ISOLATION	30
(7) ARM CIRCLES	32
(8) ABDOMINALS	34
(9) BREAST STROKE PREP	36
(10) CHILD'S POSE	38
(11) HUNDRED	40
(12) HALF ROLL BACK	43
(13) ROLL UP PREP	45
(14) SINGLE LEG CIRCLE	48
(15) SITTING SPINE TWIST	50
(16) SIDE LYING LATERAL OBLIQUES	53
(17) SINGLE LEG STRETCH PREP	55
(18) DOUBLE LEG STRETCH PREP	59
(19) SCISSORS PREP	61

(20) SHOULDER BRIDGE PREP 64
(21) ROLL OVER PREP 68
(22) DOUBLE LEG EXTENSION PREP 70
(23) SINGLE LEG KICK 73
(24) SAW 75
(25) NECK PULL PREP 78
(26) OBLIQUES ROLL BACK 81
(27) TEASER PREP 84
(28) SIDE LYING CLAM SERIES 87
(29) SIDE LEG LIFT SERIES 95
(30) CAT STRETCH 99
(31) SITTING SPINE STRETCH FORWARD 102
(32) SWAN DIVE PREP 105
(33) SWIMMING PREP 107
(34) LEG PULL FRONT PREP 110
(35) REVERSE PLANK PREP (LEG PULL) 112
(36) PILATES PUSH-UP PREP 1 115
(37) ELBOW PLANK PREP 118
(38) SLOW DOUBLE LEG STRETCH PREP 120
(39) FRONT LEG KICK 122
(40) SIDE BEND PREP 124
(41) SIDE ELBOW STRETCH WITH TWIST 128
(42) SIDE BEND WITH TWIST 130
(43) PILATES PUSH-UP PREP 2 133
(44) SEAL 139
(45) MERMAID 141

EXTRAS

REFERENCE CHART 143
GLOSSARY 144
FUNDAMENTAL MINI WORKOUTS 157
RESOURCES 163
PILATES ON THE BOSU® TEAM 165

ACKNOWLEDGMENTS

About the Author

Miriane Taylor has been teaching Pilates for over 30 years. During that time, she has been creating and teaching the Pilates mat work, as well as associated equipment, and has been creating a unique set of exercises on the BOSU based on each individual's needs.

Miriane has written many Pilates training manuals and has appeared in eight of the Stott Pilates video series as well as co-produced the video, Core Toner (Equilibrium Videos). Miriane is co-author of the "Get on it" BOSU Balance Trainer Book.

She is certified as a Pilates teacher-trainer and master instructor, and certified in the Garuda method under James D'Silva (inventor, creator and founder of the Garuda method), including the mat, apparatus and Garuda machine. Miriane is based in Toronto, Canada (www.taylor-dpilates.com) and teaches workshops both at home and internationally.

Credits

Author:	**Miriane Taylor**
Forward:	**Colleen Craig**
Models:	**Nadim Habib and Miriane Taylor**
Photography:	**Eddie Kastrau, Sana Khan, Brian Taylor**
Copy Editor:	**Carol Anderson**
Illustrations:	**Charmaine Hew Wing**
Graphic Design and Layout:	**Eddie Kastrau**
Costume Design and Build:	**Lexi Soukoreff (Daub and Design)**
Cover Model:	**Miriane Taylor**

INTRODUCTIONS

FORWARD BY COLLEEN CRAIG

Miriane Taylor's Pilates on the BOSU eBook Series

When I began my Pilates training in the late 1990s at the Toronto Stott Pilates studio, I had the great luck to meet the master teacher, Miriane Taylor. As an aspiring Pilates teacher-trainee I loved watching Miriane teach. I admired how she explained exercises and motivated her students. She is one of those rare gifted instructors who not only teaches with compassion and skill but also performs the Pilates exercises with grace and perfection.

Over the years our careers went in different directions: Miriane was busy building her Toronto studio and method, Taylor-d Pilates, appearing in best-selling videos, and writing Pilates training manuals for the international workshops she taught. She is not only certified as a Pilates teacher-trainer, but also as a teacher of the Garuda method under James D'Silva. In addition, she co-produced the video Core Toner with Equilibrium Videos.

I did not see Miriane for a couple of years, but she was the first person I called whenever I needed extra training, whether it be with small or large balls, or the BOSU-- especially when it came to the BOSU. There is simply no other teacher I know with the knowledge, creativity and passion that Miriane brings to this unique piece of equipment. In the early 2010s I was scheduled to teach a number of full-day workshops in various cities in Brazil that including not only small and large balls, but the BOSU. A BOSU was relatively new to me and I was terrified of teaching large groups of discerning Brazilian fitness professionals and Pilates teachers. Miriane spent weeks with me, preparing me for these workshops, sharing with me all that she knew. She taught me how to mount and dismount this two-sided dome, where to put my body in relation to the apex, how the flat side as well as the dome can be best utilized. The notes she gave me were crystal clear, her training had been spot on, and her voice—that unique and lovely voice—built up my confidence and reminded me again of the joy of being an enthusiastic student guided by a brilliant teacher.

The next time we connected she was about to publish a book, Get on it! BOSU Balance Trainer (written with Jane Aronovitch, and published by Ulysses Press). The BOSU was becoming very popular and already foreign rights were being negotiated. I could tell this book was going to sell well.

Miriane Taylor has now created an entirely new type of book—an interactive ebook. Pilates on the BOSU is worlds ahead of an ordinary manual or guide. Eddie Kastrau designed this gorgeous ebook with accessibility in mind. It is easy to use and full of live links that add extra information and layers to each exercise. For example, I was looking up an essential exercise on the BOSU, Breast Stroke Prep, performed by Miriane in stunning photos, and I clicked on the word 'abdominals'. I was transported to a page of striking anatomical illustrations, by Charmaine Hew Wing. I knew then that all of Miriane's hard work, and years of persevering had paid off.

Pilates on the BOSU consists of three ebooks. The first book is called: Pilates on the BOSU: Fundamentals. Many of the essential Pilates mat exercises are enhanced by use of the BOSU. Miriane establishes the goals of each exercise, which muscles are working, and then moves on to explain how the unique features of the BOSU enhances the movement. Miriane is also extremely skilled in using the BOSU for beginners; many modifications are shown that will be useful for physiotherapists and people recovering from injuries. The second book is an Intermediate level, called: Pilates on the BOSU: Intermediate, and it builds on the fundamentals to show many more challenging Pilate's-based exercises for athletes, dancers, gym enthusiasts and even older adults (or other age groups) who are getting back into exercise for strength, balance and core. The third book, Pilates on the BOSU: Advanced, puts the BOSU on steroids and creates a fun and playful way to build strength, stability and confidence.

This ground-breaking, comprehensive guide is a must-have resource for Pilates and other fitness professionals, and anyone wanting to learn how to use this two-sided dome to enhance any workout. I want to express my gratitude to all that Miriane has shared with me. Congratulations on Pilates on the BOSU eBook series !

-Colleen Craig
Founder of Pilates on the Ball
www.pilatesontheball.com

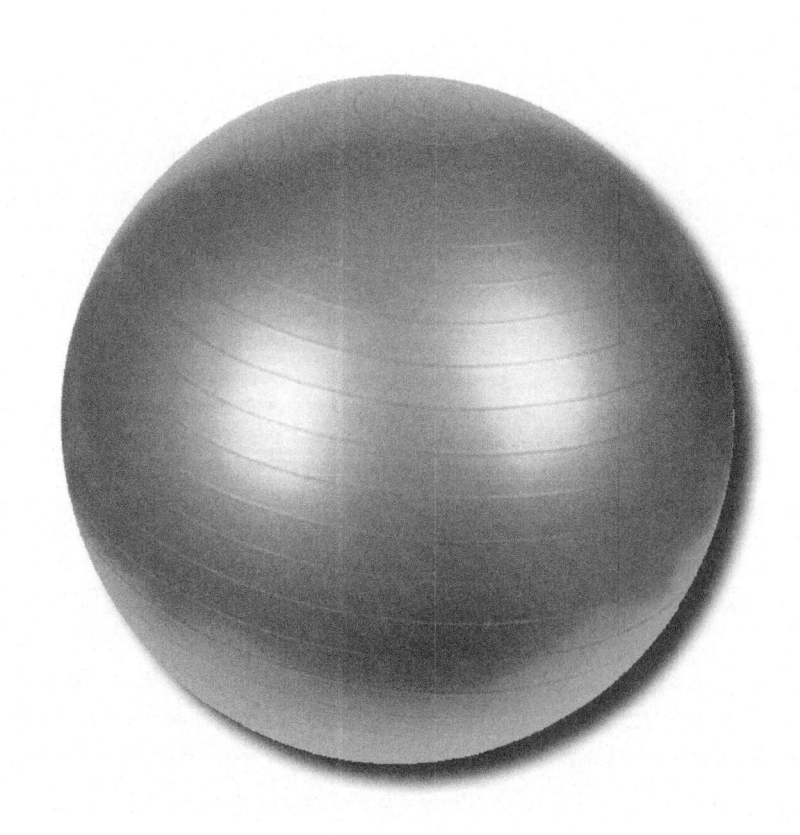

MY BOSU® JOURNEY

My journey on the BOSU began in 2002 when I was first introduced to it.

At first, just standing on the dome felt like an impossible task. It took a good few days to master standing on it, never mind stepping up and stepping down or moving on and off the BOSU (like working out in a step class.) I thought to myself "How very clever...taking a Fitness Ball and cutting it in half. Brilliant."

Before then, I'd only known about equipment such as the Balance Board and the Wobble Disk for supporting balance, control and equilibrium in the body. During the two years from 2000 to 2002, I was teaching in South Africa, and spent quite a bit of time working with my physiotherapist friend Daryl Kruger, who loved the Fitness Ball (aka Fit Ball, Big Ball, Exercise Ball, Stability Ball, etc.). He showed me new and innovative ways to use the Fitness Ball, as well as how to use it with clients.

Every day during a week long beach holiday, we practiced trying to stand on the Fitness Ball... Hopeless! But really fun, especially since you can place the ball in the sand and create a little hollow for the Fitness Ball to sit in. We tried over and over again to stand on the Fitness Ball or jump from two feet and land on the Ball, but the best we could do was kneel on it. We talked about the muscles we should be using and how to activate the core during each movement in order to master moving on and off the Ball. The Fitness Ball was/is clever and brilliant if you know how to use it without falling and hurting yourself, as explored by the Swiss fitness professionals who greatly expanded ways of using the Ball.

Kneeling was easily mastered, but standing was another story. We practiced for the entire week; we might balance for an instant and then would fall in the sand. Settling into sand to practice is your best bet, since practicing standing on the Fitness Ball on hard surfaces can be dangerous.

Daryl shared some of the videos he had acquired from Swiss practitioners that showed AMAZING, seemingly impossible ways to use the Fitness Ball. I marveled at their ability to use the Fitness Ball in such creative and mind blowing ways. Simply fantastic!!!! The Fitness Ball does offer endless possibilities, as you can discover in Colleen Craig's "Pilates on the Ball", "Abs on the Ball" and "Strength Training on the Ball."

I continued to study and use the Fitness Ball in my Pilates Mat Work classes. I started getting people to use the Fitness Ball sitting at their desks to help with proper posture and strong legs. The Fitness Ball was magical.

Then the **BOSU** was introduced to me by Deidre Pretlove, an accomplished tri-athlete, and a physiotherapist at Toronto's Personal Best Physiotherapy Clinic. At first, I was bewildered, and the **BOSU** seemed rather intimidating. It took me awhile to understand its mechanics. I became intrigued, then awed and absorbed – I fell in love with this piece of equipment and started to dig deeper into understanding its purpose. I wanted to understand what it was all about.

The **BOSU** Ball was born in 2000, created by Californian David Weck. This clever piece of equipment has kept me on my toes and allowed me to take the Pilates Mat Work to whole new level. To my

FUNDAMENTALS

surprise, my biggest CHALLENGE was getting on and standing on the dome. I practiced every single day and kept notes. I discovered that I was not using my core correctly! I danced professionally for several years, and now I was having trouble balancing on top of the **BOSU**. This was a bit confusing.

I determined to learn as much as I could by studying anatomy, understanding the muscles that stabilize and control the core, and those that flex and extend the spine. Every aspect of the **BOSU** in relation to the body was fascinating to me. Through this learning process I discovered the full benefit of the **BOSU** and how EVERYONE can gain more strength, and stretch and tone muscles while working "smarter not harder".

I studied every single video that David Weck and his **BOSU** team created. This study further intrigued and excited me, as I grew to understand that the **BOSU** has SO MUCH more to offer people than meets the eye. Whether you are sitting at your desk, walking, running, or standing all day, the **BOSU** is for you.

I gathered all this information and ran with it. I created a course I called "Pilates on the **BOSU**, incorporating all Pilates Mat exercises on the dome". At first the material I developed seemed enough for one book. Thanks go to Colleen Craig, who advised me that there was actually enough material for three books.

These books have several intentions. First, to encourage your motivation to build a better, stronger body. Second, to develop belief in yourself as you become more balanced. Third, to support understanding of your strengths and weaknesses, and become more confident and toned.

Videos will follow these books.

While you adapt to the surface of the **BOSU**, the core muscles are challenged but in a controlled space. The space around you should be wide and long enough so that you can really own your space. Having fun using the full **BOSU** and getting as much out of the surface around you and on top of the dome is crucial. This will assist you in all avenues of life, whether you sit, walk a lot, or are an athlete. Working with the **BOSU** helps ensure that your Pilates Mat Work will become far more enjoyable.

The Pilates Mat Work can be a strain on the neck muscles and perhaps even on the back. Using the unstable surface of the dome gives you the opportunity to learn how to negotiate the surface and adapt the surface to your physical needs.

The intention of the Fundamental Level is to become aware of and lessen any stress or strain on your neck, back or shoulders. You will learn how to execute each exercise with pure precision and control. You will develop a sense of control, of owning the **BOSU** and the surface around you, rather than the surface of the **BOSU** owning you.

My hope is to inspire you to develop your own creativity to use the **BOSU** in the best way you can, and even create your own fun on top of the dome.

PARTS OF THE BOSU®

TOP VIEW - DOME SIDE

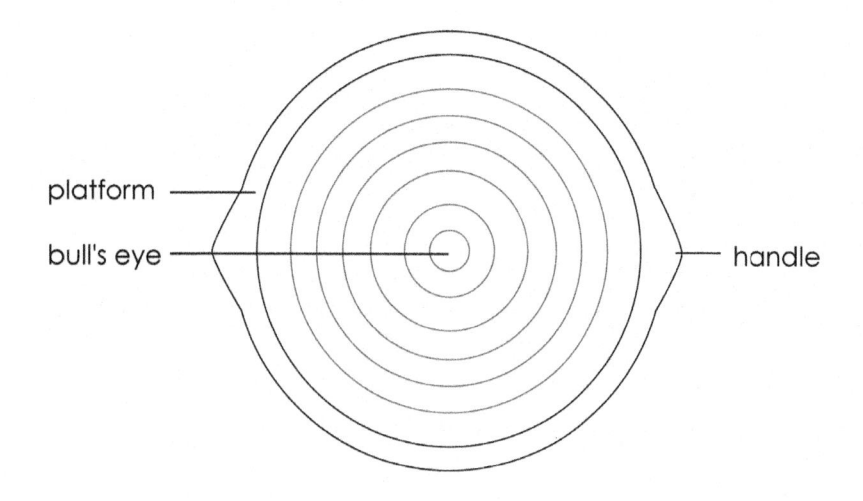

- platform
- bull's eye
- handle

BOTTOM VIEW - FLAT SIDE

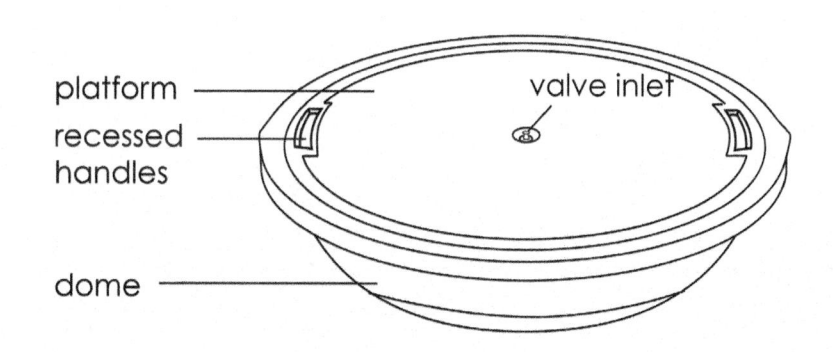

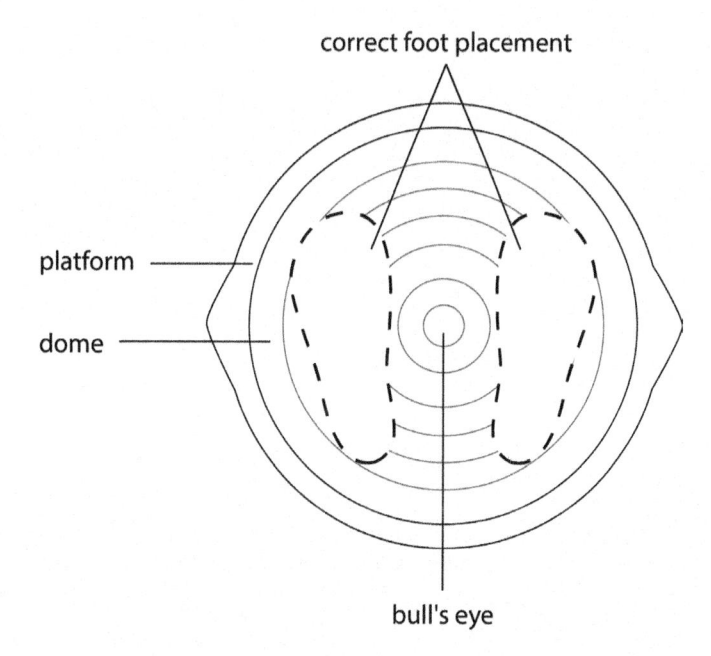

- platform
- recessed handles
- dome
- valve inlet

- correct foot placement
- platform
- dome
- bull's eye

FUNDAMENTALS

WHAT IS A BOSU®?

Short for 'both sides up' the **BOSU** Balance Trainer®, or **BOSU** (pronounced 'Bo' like the boy's name, and 'Sue' like the girl's name), was invented by Californian David Weck in 1999 and launched in 2000. Since then it has become one of the most popular fitness tools in the industry.

The **BOSU** is approximately 25 inches wide and looks like a big exercise ball that's cut in half. One side is dome-shaped; the other is flat. The dome side is inflatable and should be filled until it is fairly firm and about 8 to 10 inches high.

As a result of its ingenious construction, the **BOSU** has two unstable surfaces that transform even the simplest moves into a fun and challenging workout. Working on an uneven surface tests your balance and forces you to use and strengthen deep core and stabilizing muscles—muscles that conventional exercise programs often miss.

Suitable for all ages and fitness levels, the **BOSU** can be used at home or in studio or gym classes. Trainers, athletes, dancers, and general fitness buffs alike use the **BOSU** to build strength and agility, tone and sculpt muscles, improve aerobic conditioning, burn fat and improve posture and alignment. The **BOSU** is also a great tool for stretching, and for incorporating Pilates Mat exercises for added challenge and proprioception.

The **BOSU** can help you trim down your waistline. Using the **BOSU** you can also combine aerobic and cardiovascular exercises with strength training, balance challenges, and flexibility—all the ingredients of a well-rounded exercise regimen.

WHY PILATES ON THE BOSU®

My own teaching principle: Taylor'd Pilates, is a comprehensive conditioning technique and can enhance performance in any activity. It will challenge co-ordination, massage internal organs, stimulate your immune system, oxygenate tissues (through the focused breathing patterns) and relax your mind. Many benefits await the committed Pilates enthusiast in a uniquely gentle, low joint stress approach to mind-body health.

It is the long-term intention of Taylor'd Pilates to make this wonderful movement experience accessible to all. We personalize the method for the individual by providing many progressions of the original work of Joseph Pilates. We aim to make a difference in elite sport performance, health, physical therapy, hospitals, exercise facilities and your own home.

The following exercises are Pilate's-based Mat Work on the **BOSU**, designed to balance musculoskeletal strength and flexibility in a holistic manner. The movements promote optimal neuromuscular patterns that are present in a normal, healthy posture and efficient movement.

The techniques work from the inside out (i.e. core musculature), rather than focusing on the superficial muscle groups alone. Many of the deep-lying core muscles have a protective function for the lumbar spine, and this may contribute to the therapeutic benefit of Pilates on the **BOSU**.

This guide is designed for Certified Pilates instructors, trainees, fitness professionals and anyone who wants to challenge their body in this unique commitment to integrating use of the **BOSU**, which on its own, is demanding and fun.

THE 6 ORIGINAL PRINCIPLES OF PILATES TRAINING

1. Concentration
2. Centering
3. Control
4. Breathing
5. Precision
6. Flowing Movement

THE 6 TAYLOR'D PILATES PRINCIPLES

1. Breathing

Breathing has an effect on many systems of the body besides the obvious mechanical effect in respiration. It is an extraordinary symphony of both powerful and subtle movement that massages internal organs, mobilizes joints, and tones and relaxes muscles.

During exercise, breathing helps to initiate the contraction of stabilizing abdominal muscles while it prevents unnecessary tension in other areas of the body. The diaphragm (primary breathing muscle) moves down during inspiration, allowing the rib cage to expand to the back and sides as much as possible.

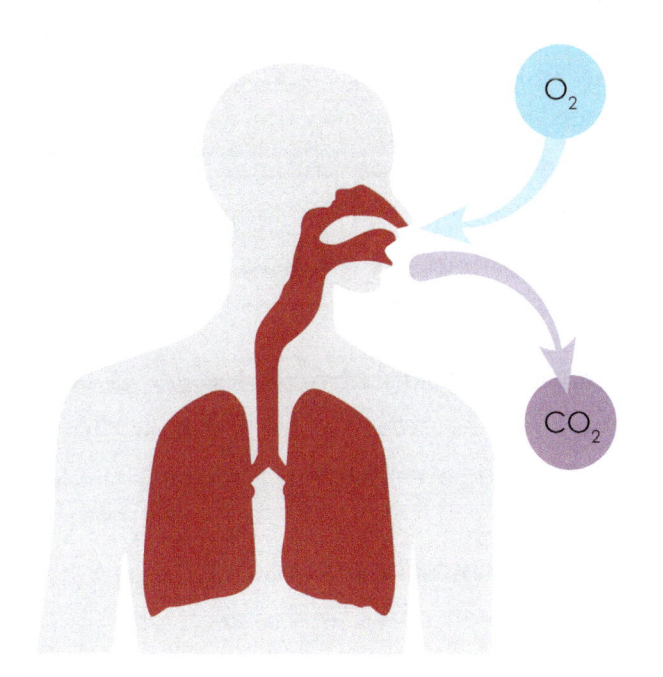

This is sometimes referred to as "thoracic breathing". Functionally, the spine extends with inspiration and during expiration the spine flexes and the ribs roll slightly forward and downward.

Using the surface of the **BOSU**, one is acutely aware of the tactile feeling on the back or stomach during breathing, feeling the ribs expand and contract against this surface.

FUNDAMENTALS

2. The Rib Cage

Lying supine, become aware of sliding the rib cage down toward the hip bones. Expiration assists in engaging the obliques (particularly the internal abdominal obliques) to create this connection between the ribs and the hips.

Awareness of the rib cage is equally important in sitting, kneeling and standing.

Using the round side of the **BOSU** provides more feedback, especially laterally to enable control and stability of the spine. The **BOSU** forces one to connect the deeper core muscles that help to contain the rib cage by simultaneously dropping and lengthening the spine. The deep core muscles are progressively challenged when sitting on the front half of the **BOSU** or having the full torso on the top of the dome.

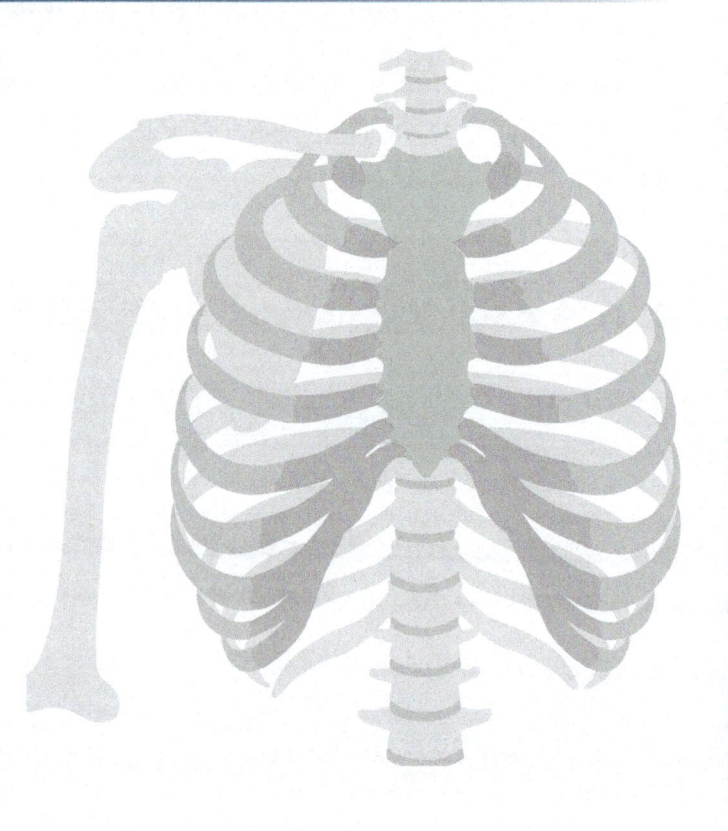

3. The Pelvic Girdle

The pelvis is located in a strategic position in the human anatomy, linking the torso with the lower extremities. This means that the pelvis co-operates with the movements of all these related structures but also contributes toward stability of the whole body.

In normal standing posture, the pelvis adapts to distribute the load of the upper body equally over both legs. When standing on one leg, other fine adjustments are required to transmit the load and still maintain a balance of the whole body. Primary movements of the spine create secondary movements of the pelvis that are linked to those of the spine and sometimes the legs.

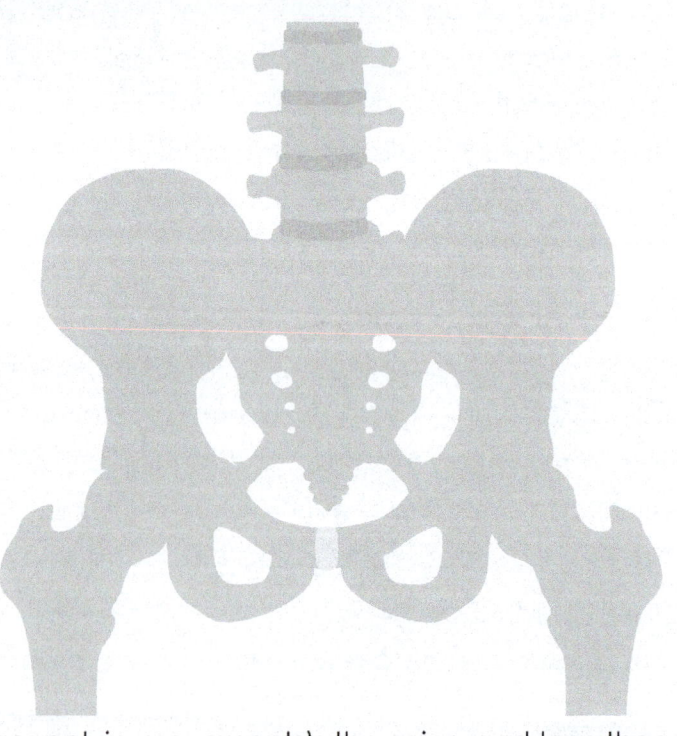

Movement can also be initiated at the pelvis (primary pelvic movements); the spine and legs then co-operate with secondary movements. Fat deposition, muscular hypertrophy and unusual sacral shapes can mislead an observer trying to judge the orientation of a subject's pelvis. Remember that skeletal alignment does not always correspond with superficial contours of the lower back. Neutral

INTRODUCTIONS

Pelvic Position – L and R anterior superior iliac spines (ASIS) and the pubic symphysis lie on the same cardinal plane. Forces around the lumbar spine are most balanced in this position and stabilization and movement potential is optimal. Due to individual variability this "position" should strictly be referred to as a range.

Neutral Spine – the normal curve of the spine that includes a normal lumbar lordosis. The apex of the curve is most commonly located at L3.

Imprinted Spine – when exercising supine with feet off the mat, facilitate spinal stabilization by slightly posteriorly tilting the pelvis, flattening the lumbar curve and allowing the spinous processes of the lumbar vertebrae to gently touch the mat. More conditioned individuals can eventually dynamically stabilize in a neutral pelvic position.

Effective lumbar stabilization is achieved through a co-contraction of the transverse abdominus and multifidi muscles. The internal abdominal obliques maintain the connection between the rib cage and the pelvic girdle.

The **BOSU** encourages tightening the deeper pelvic floor muscles, and indirectly affects some of the core muscles in the back, helping us to keep the pelvis more connected, especially when standing on top of the dome. Practicing to stabilize on this unstable surface helps us to recruit the muscle stabilizers that help to make the spine move safely and effectively.

The internal abdominal obliques help to stabilize the hips. The transverse abdominus help to stabilize the pelvis.

4. The Scapulae

Each scapula should move in a smooth and co-ordinated relationship with the shoulder joints (scapula-humeral rhythm).

Avoid forcing the scapulae down, elevating or rounding the shoulders or winging the scapulae.

Scapulae stabilizers (collectively referred to as scapular stabilizers), include:

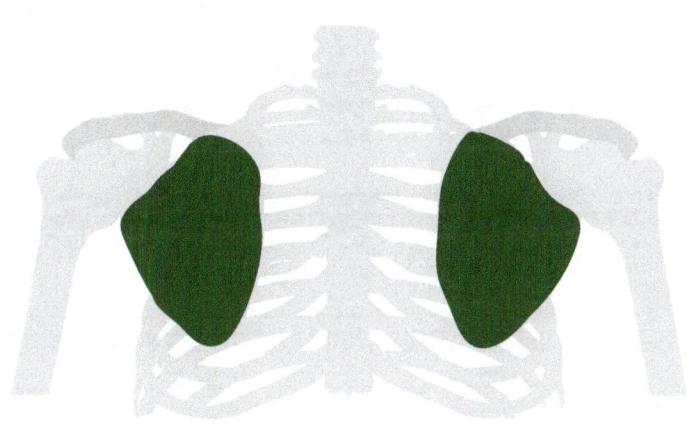

- Trapezius muscle (upper and lower fibers)
- Levator scapulae
- Rhomboid major and minor
- Serratus anterior
- Pectoralis minor

FUNDAMENTALS 13

In sitting and rolling through the back while on the **BOSU**, where the spine is working and the arms are being used for balance, the shoulder blade muscles are consistently engaged. Optimal body alignment is all about nurturing a stress-free state when you exercise. This is especially evident in the awareness of the neck and shoulder muscles, which tend to tighten under stress.

5. Head and Cervical Spine

While exercising in supine, avoid developing neck tension while the head is lifted off the mat. When the upper body is flexed off the mat, the cervical spine should maintain the same line as the thoracic spine.

Avoid jamming the chin into the chest or protruding the chin forward.

Before flexing the upper body off the mat, stretch the back of the neck to create a lengthening of the cervical spine (like a small nodding movement).

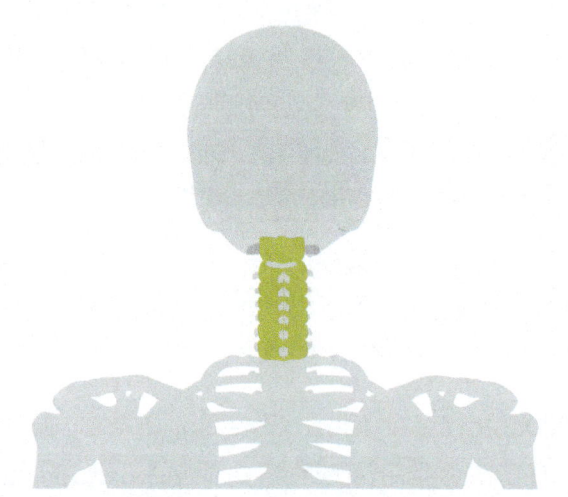

To save the body from stressing or straining, hands behind the head are preferred. Using the surface of the **BOSU** when lying down with the torso along the mat supports the weight of the head, especially in someone who is hunched in the upper spine. This support includes elongating or lengthening the spine to improve the neutrality of the head and cervical spine muscles.

6. Feet and Ankles

It is important to maintain alignment of weight-bearing structures and to distribute the body weight evenly over the supportive surface area of the feet.

When flexing at the knee joints, the mid-lines of the patellae normally track in the same vertical plane as the space between the 2nd and 3rd toes.

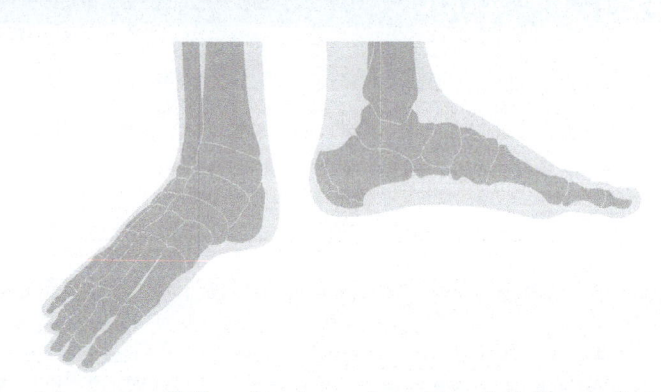

Practicing to stabilize on this unstable surface helps us to recruit the feet and ankle stabilizers that help with balance and control. Proper placement of the feet, whether sitting on the floor or standing on the **BOSU**, will activate the leg muscles, building more strength and flexibility in the feet and ankles. We often forget about the feet muscles, and the **BOSU** is an essential tool that helps to constantly remind us to engage the feet and ankles.

PRACTICING SAFE BOSU®

One of the best things about the **BOSU** is that it is very easy to mount and dismount, whether you are sitting, standing or kneeling. If you lose your balance at any point, simply step off or make yourself comfortable and start over when you're ready. As with any piece of exercise equipment, however, it pays to be careful.

While using the **BOSU** during your workout it is important to place the **BOSU** on a yoga mat; this way when your feet are placed on the floor you won't slip or slide. Keep a towel handy to wipe down any perspiration while doing your workout. The space around you should be that of at least 3 yoga mats placed side by side. With this amount of space around you, you can easily circle your arms wide without any obstacles in the way.

Inflate the dome until it is firm. The flat side of the **BOSU** is a solid platform about 25 inches wide. The handles on either side make it easy to hold or grip.

Store your **BOSU** in a shaded area away from any heated surface. For a longer life, keep the **BOSU** surface clean at all times and wear shoes that you use indoors only. Do not wear socks. Socks could stick on the dome and you could injure yourself.

Transitions between exercises are as important as the exercises themselves. When flowing from one exercise to another, perform transitions with equal care and attention. Starting positions also need meticulous attention, whether you are standing, sitting, kneeling, or balancing on the **BOSU**. When mounting the **BOSU**, during any exercise where your hips are on top of the dome, it is important to ease yourself carefully toward the mat into inversion (head and shoulder on mat) to avoid lower back and neck strain.

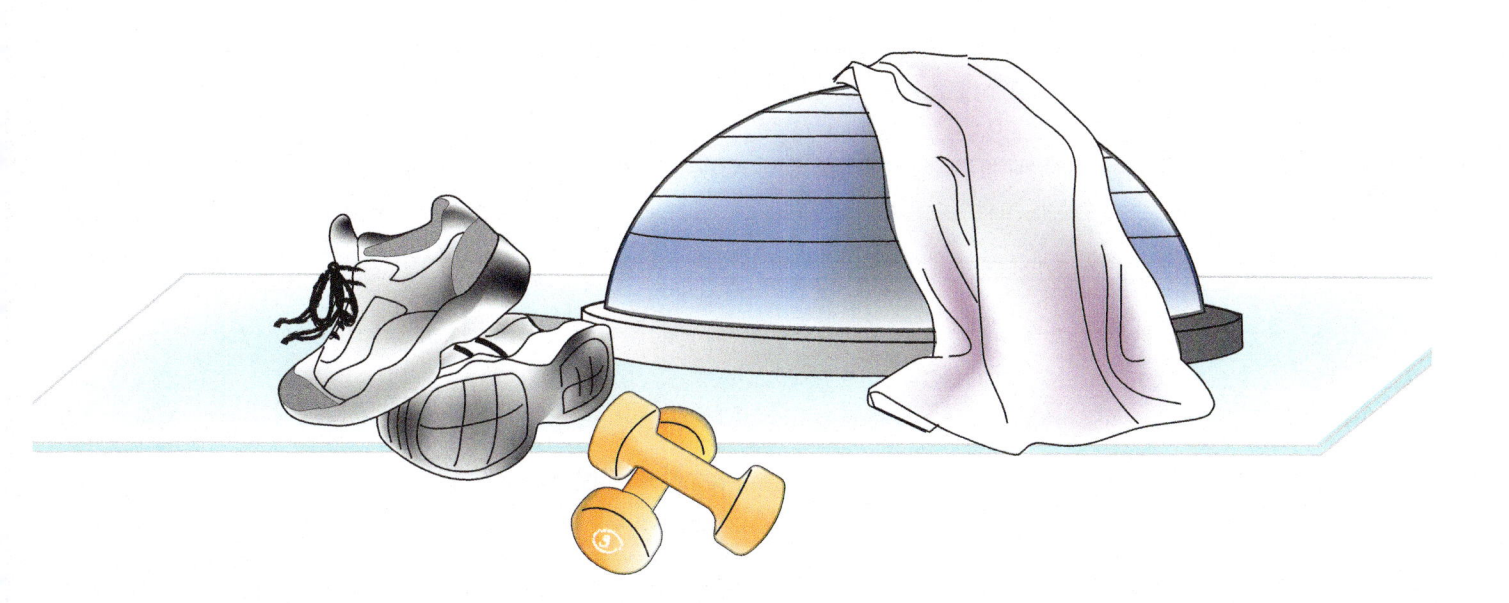

FUNDAMENTALS

ADVANTAGES OF USING THE BOSU®

- Tones and strengthens the entire body.
- Targets deep and superficial muscles.
- Adds resistance and weight-bearing to your workout.
- Works the body as a unit in an integrated way.
- Provides a good base for functional, cardiovascular and strength training.
- Allows us to work through a full range of motion and multiple planes of movement - rotating our limbs in and out, in circles and diagonals, bringing them across the mid-line, etc.
- Trains the muscles to work together, encouraging cross- and inter-connections.
- Improves balance, control and co-ordination.
- Offers a fun and dynamic way to work out.

PILATES APPROACH TO USING THE BOSU® BENEFITS

- Enhances co-ordination and improves posture.
- Increases flexibility and movement confidence.
- Encourages sensory motor feedback.
- Supports renewed sense of body awareness and body positioning.
- Promotes mindful training in the full body.
- Elongates muscles and improves muscle tone.
- Can boost movement performance and efficiency.
- Integrates stabilizers and counter-balance forces.
- Improves proprioception, balance and control.

LAYOUT OF THE EXERCISES

Throughout the books, you will find Modifications which are designed to accompany the exercise and provide alternate variations to allow you to go deeper or simplify the underlying exercise.

The three levels of Modifications are:

1) ASSIST: Suggestions as to how to make the exercise safer and/or easier on the body.
2) SIMPLIFY: To make the exercise easier to execute.
3) CHALLENGE: To make the exercise more difficult to execute.

Below each exercise you will also find a section titled: **MUSCULAR INTENTION**, which describes which muscle groups are being targeting in the exercise.

And finally, with each exercise you will find helpful **TIPS** to assist you in finding the ideal placement to maximize the effective of each exercise.

DESCRIPTION OF THE FUNDAMENTAL LEVEL

Carefully designed progressions allow anyone to learn the fundamental nature of the Fundamental exercises before more complex and challenging repertoire is mastered. Fundamental Level exercises can be executed so that the **BOSU** is used for extra support in the Pilates Mat Work, in particular with neck and shoulder tension. The **BOSU** can also be used to assist in movement. In many cases the exercises can be varied to support or simplify movement, or to challenge the practitioner's co-ordination, strength, balance and flexibility.

One of the basic principles of the Fundamental Level is the placement of the body in relation to the **BOSU**. For example, the **Abdominal Prep** exercise is first done with the head on the dome and the torso along the mat. (picture 1) This placement supports the head and neck as the neck muscles grow progressively stronger. Sitting higher up against the **BOSU** on the mat, with the back ribs against the front half of the dome (picture 2) will facilitate a fuller extension and flexion of the spine. The head and neck are supported by placing the hands behind the head. For someone who is experiencing kyphosis (round upper back), this position is the perfect place to do the **Abdominal Prep** until the upper spine has achieved increased mobility. This is an exceptional way to support the neck and build strength in the upper spine.

ABDOMINAL PREP

picture 1   picture 2

FUNDAMENTALS

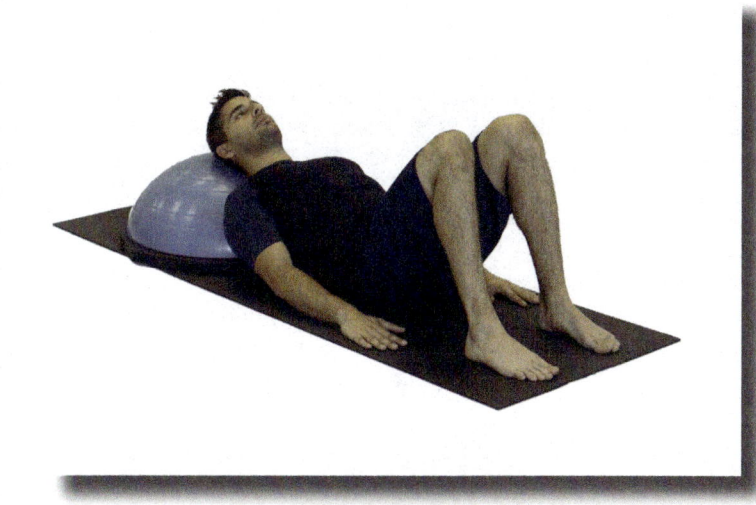

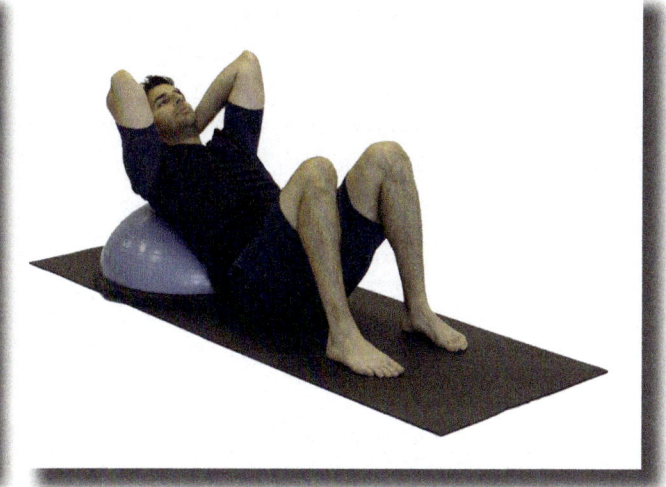

PILATES ON THE BOSU

FUNDAMENTALS

EXERCISES

"Success is the sum of small efforts, repeated day in and day out."

-- Robert J. Collier

(1) SPINAL MOBILIZATION

Start Position

1. Spine neutral.
2. Sitting in front of the BOSU on the mat.
3. Thoracic and lumbar spine resting against the front half of dome.
4. Hands clasped behind the head, elbows reaching toward the ceiling.
5. Knees bent slightly apart and parallel, feet on the mat and in-line with sitting bones.

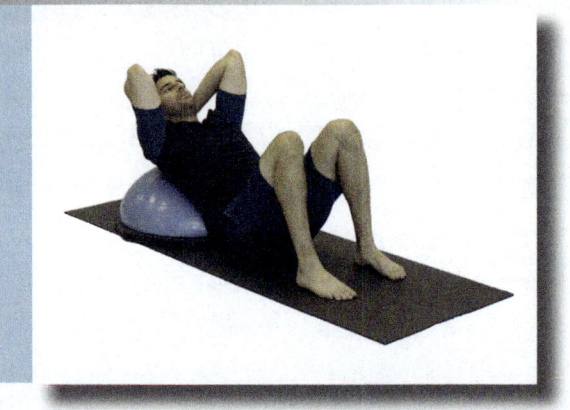

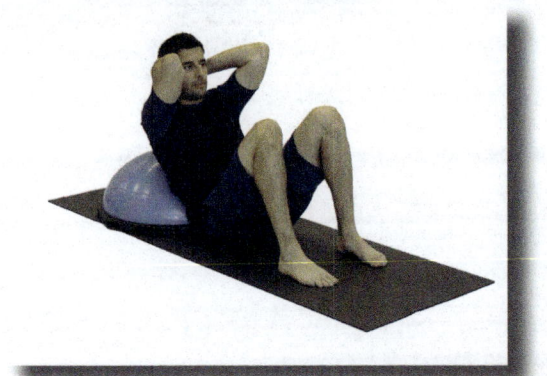

Upper Spine Mobilization

Inhale	Extend the upper spine toward the back wall, reaching the elbows to where the wall and the ceiling meet.
Exhale	Slide the ribs toward the hips, curling the upper body forward while reaching the elbows toward the ceiling.
Reps	X5

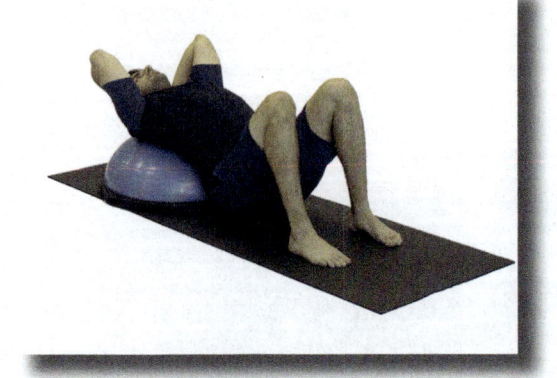

18   **EXERCISES**

Lower Spine Mobilization

Inhale   To prepare

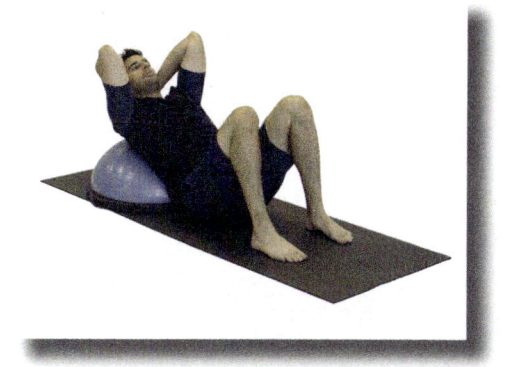

Exhale   Curl or scoop the tailbone off the mat.

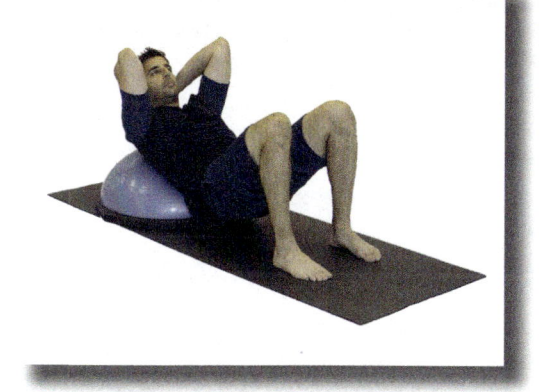

Inhale   Place the tailbone back onto the mat.
Exhale   Return to **Start Position**.
Reps   X5

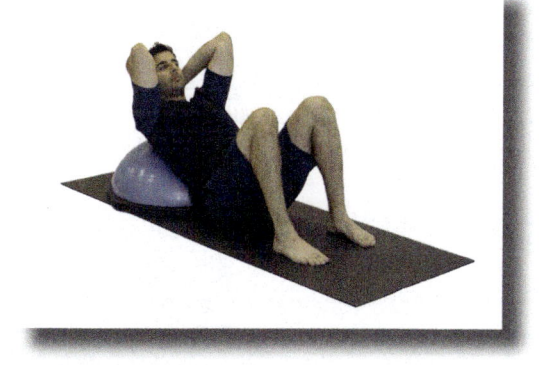

Full Spine Mobilization

Inhale   Extend the spine, while the hips stay on the mat.

FUNDAMENTALS   19

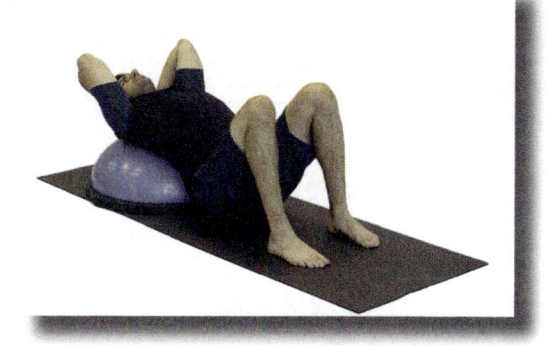

Exhale   Curl the upper body forward, simultaneously curling the lower body off the mat.

Reps   X5

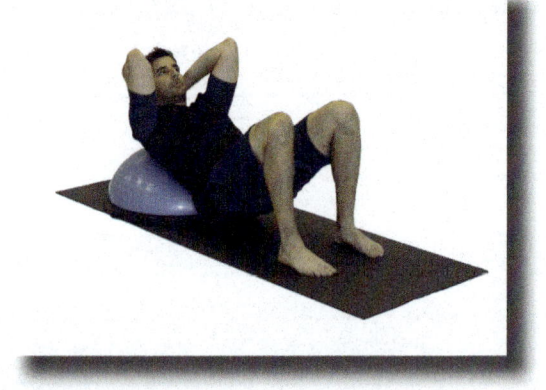

Modified

1. Start in extension. Legs straight, feet flexed, slightly apart or together, hips down. Curl the upper body only. Reps X5 (SIMPLIFY)

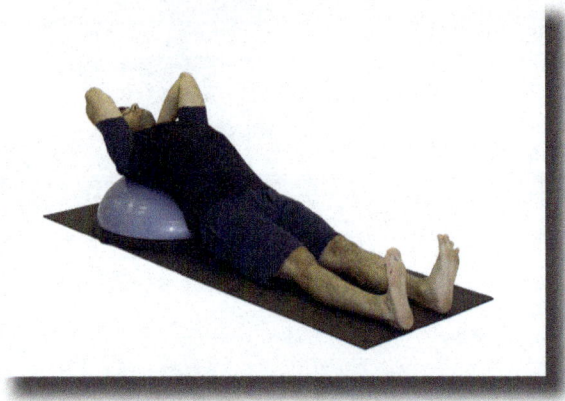

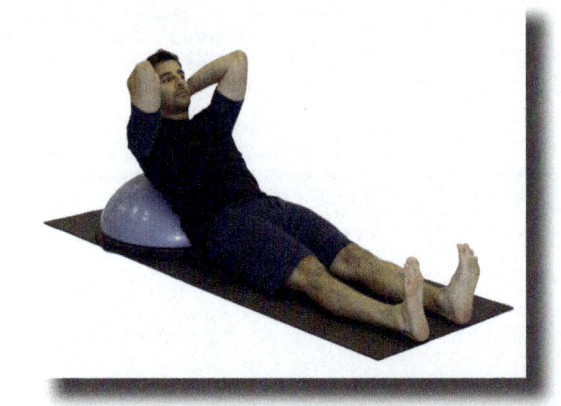

2. Start in the curl forward and lift the hips as you extend the spine backward, legs straight. Reps X5 (CHALLENGE)

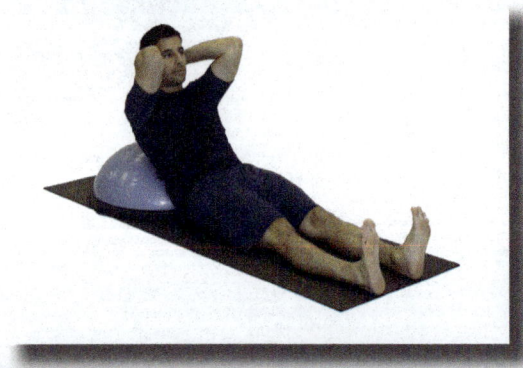

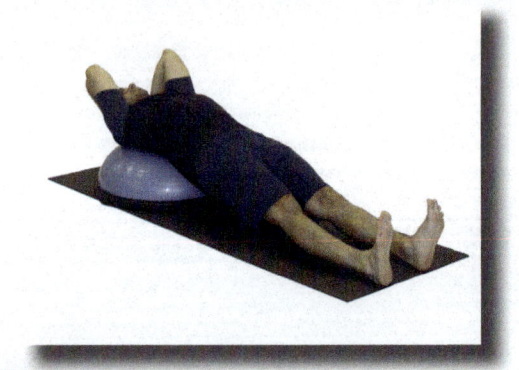

Muscular Intention

- Releasing and mobilizing the full spine
- Connecting to the deep abdominals during forward flexion and the paraspinals and glutes in extension.

Tips

✔ Cradle the head in the hands to lengthen the neck,
✔ Slide the shoulders down the back and simultaneously press the head into the hands to lengthen the neck.
✔ Reaching the elbows toward the ceiling.
✔ Lengthen the back of the legs, reaching through both heels.

(2) HIP RELEASE

Start Position

1. Spine neutral.
2. Head and shoulders on dome.
3. Collar bones wide.
4. Palms down with hands along mat, reaching toward feet.
5. Knees bent slightly apart and parallel.
6. Feet on the mat and in-line with sitting bones.
7. Hips on the mat.

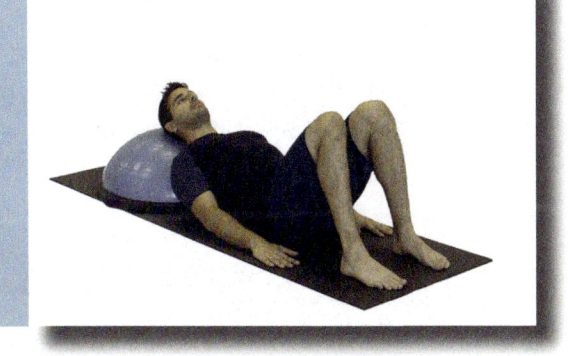

Exercise

Inhale	To prepare.
Exhale	Squeeze the lower glutes and slightly lift the hips off the mat.
Inhale	Release the squeeze of the lower glutes, place the hips back on the mat.
Reps	X5

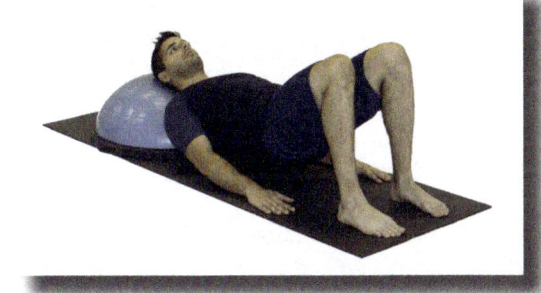

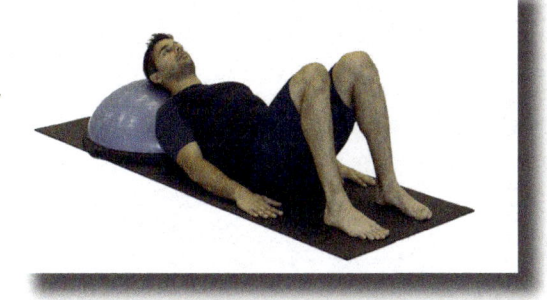

3. Head, shoulders and spine along the mat, legs overtop of the BOSU. Squeeze the glutes and press the back of the legs into the dome, as you lift the hips. Reps X5 (SIMPLIFY)

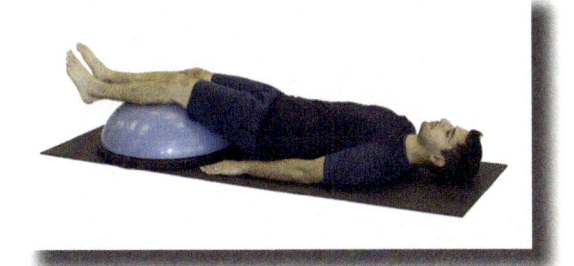

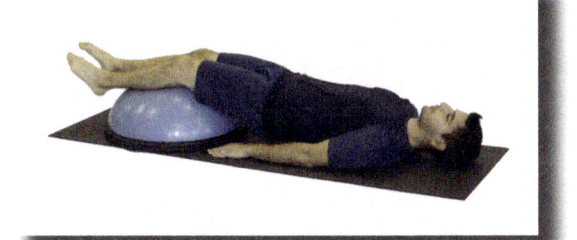

FUNDAMENTALS 21

Modified

1. Press both feet into the dome, then squeeze and release the glutes. Reps X5 (SIMPLIFY)

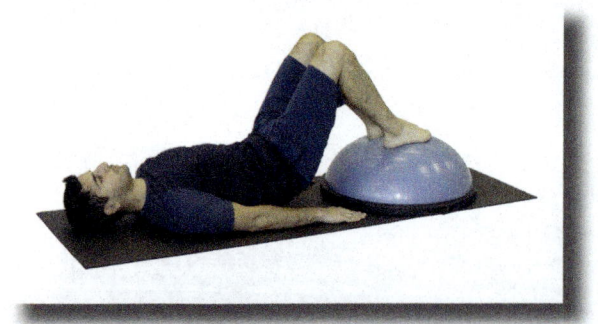

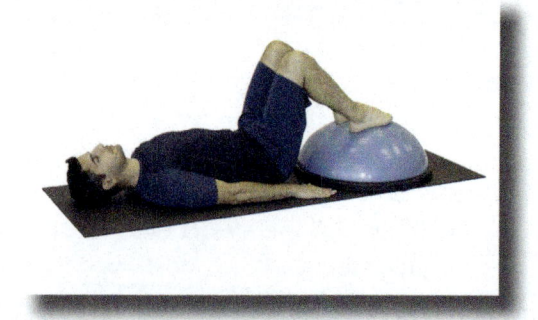

Muscular Intention

- Engaging the glutes and hamstrings, while releasing the hip flexors.
- Working the lower abdominals.
- Working the rhomboids, latissimus dorsi and triceps, pressing the arms into the mat.

Tips

- ✔ Relax the quadriceps.
- ✔ Maintain fluidity during the pelvic tilt and glute squeeze.
- ✔ Slide the shoulders down the back to lengthen the neck.
- ✔ Keep the feet and knees in line with sitting bones.
- ✔ Press the arms into the mat.

(3) ARCH AND CURL SPINE

Start Position

1. Spine neutral.
2. Sitting in front of the BOSU.
3. Hands clasped behind the head, elbows reaching toward the ceiling.
4. Knees bent slightly apart and parallel.
5. Feet on the mat and in-line with sitting bones.
6. Hips on the mat.

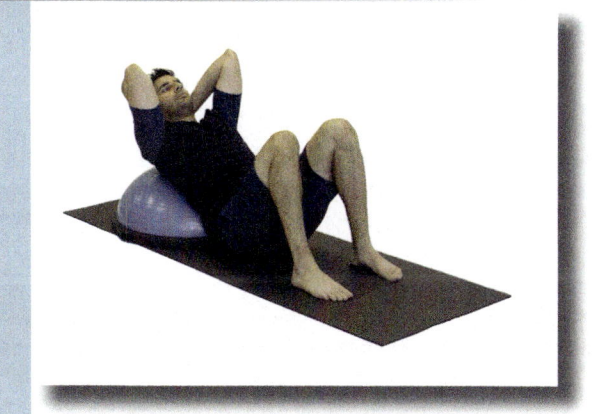

Exercise

Inhale   Extend the spine further back.

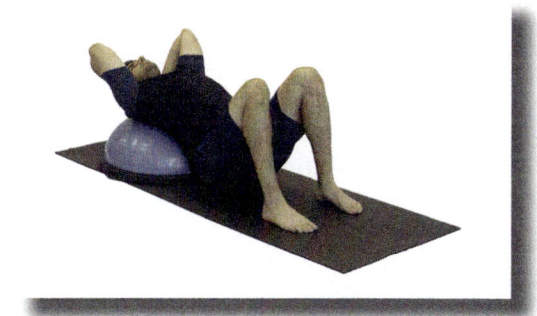

Exhale   Curl the upper body forward, Squeeze the lower glutes to lift the hips off the mat. Lead with the tailbone on the way up.

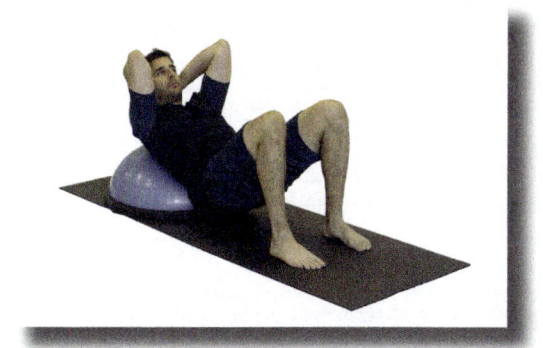

Inhale   To release the lower glutes, lower the hips back on the mat. Lead with the pubic bone on the way down. Simultaneously, extend the spine back to an arch.

Reps   X5

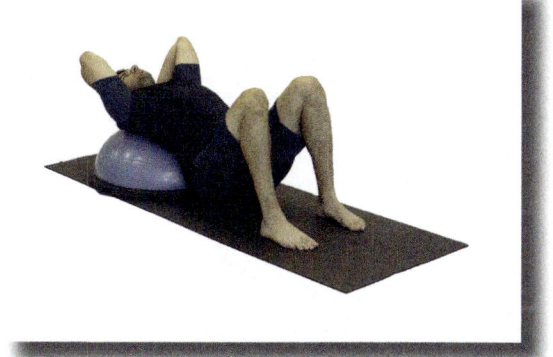

FUNDAMENTALS

Modified

1. Head and shoulders on the dome. Lengthen the lower spine along the mat. Hands on the hips. Squeeze and release the lower glutes. (Practice tailbone leads the way up and pubic bone leads the way down to the mat).
Reps X10 (SIMPLIFY)

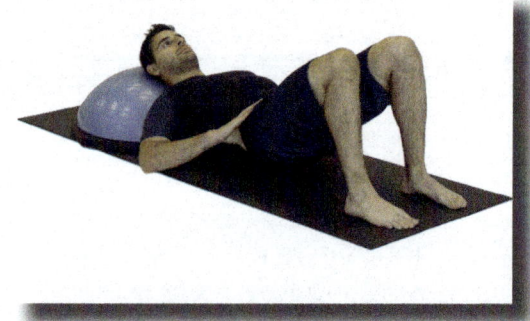

2. Feet on the dome. Press feet down onto the dome and squeeze the lower glutes. Tailbone leads the way up. Pubic bone leads the way down. Reps X10 (SIMPLIFY)

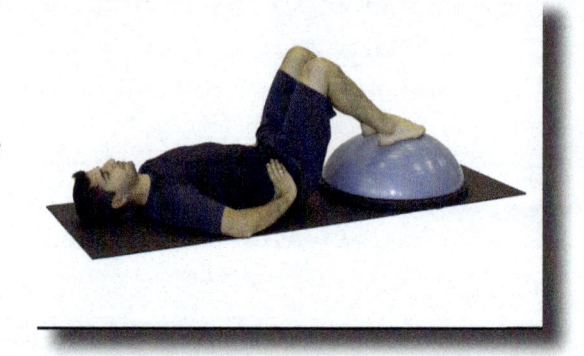

Muscular Intention

- Connecting the lower glutes and hamstrings, while releasing the hip flexors.
- Freeing the lower spine while working the back extensors and lower abdominals.

Tips

✔ Relax the quadriceps.
✔ Maintain fluidity during the pelvic tilt and release.
✔ Slide the shoulders down the back to lengthen the back of the neck.
✔ Keep the feet and knees in line with sitting bones.
✔ Keep the inner thighs connected with feet on the dome.

(4) CIRCLE UPPER BODY

Start Position

1. Spine neutral.
2. Sitting in front of the BOSU with spine extended.
3. Hands clasped behind the head, elbows reaching toward the ceiling.
4. Knees bent slightly apart and parallel.
5. Feet on the mat and in-line with sitting bones.
6. Hips on the mat.

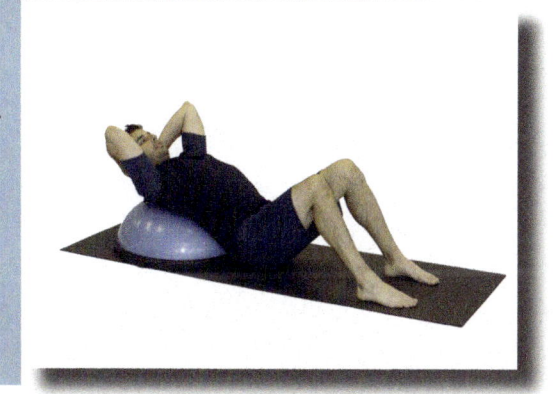

Exercise

Inhale   Lean upper body to the R, opening the L ribs.

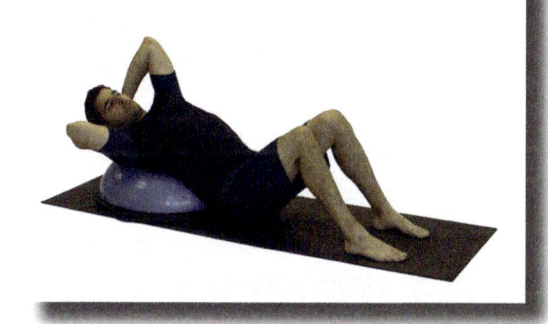

Exhale   Connecting the R rib to the R hip, then connect the L rib to the L hip. Body is curled forward.

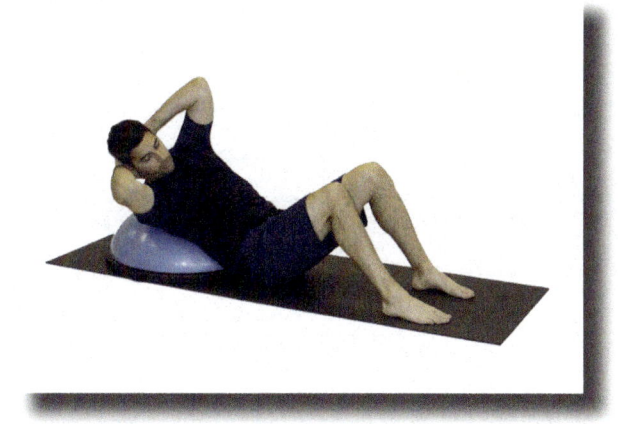

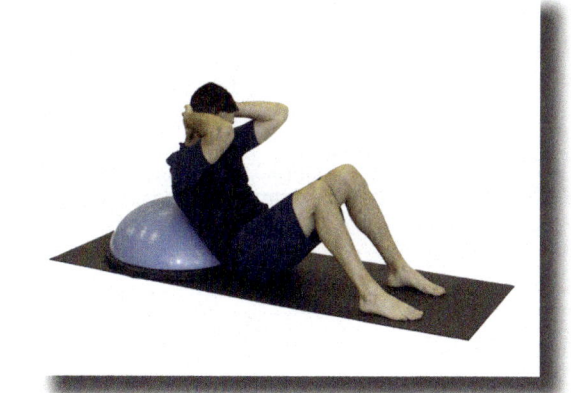

FUNDAMENTALS 25

Inhale   As you lean to the L, open the R ribs.

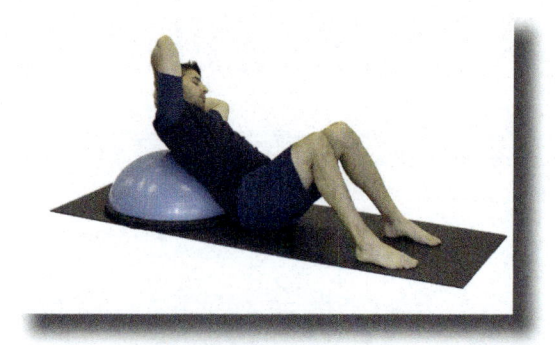

Exhale   Then opening both ribs as you extend the spine back with elbows reaching back. Continue the circle toward the R.

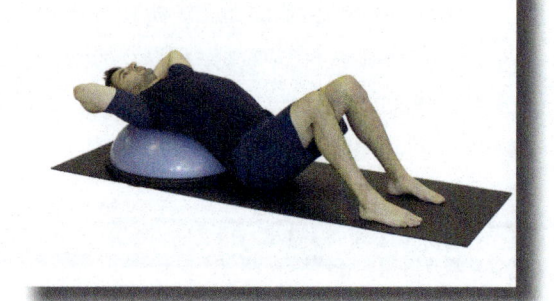

Reps   X5 R/L

Modified

1. Lean to the R side of dome and open the L ribs, then lean to the L side of dome and open the R ribs, no circle. Reps X3-5 R/L (SIMPLIFY)

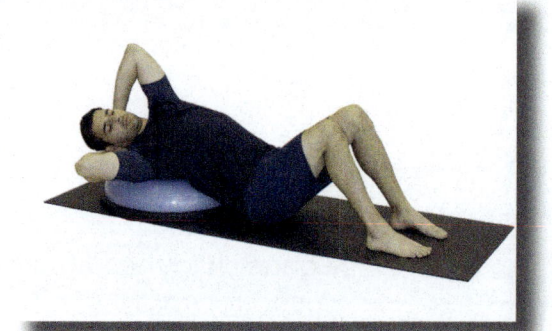

2. Opening the lateral rib cage and extend L arm. Reps X5 R/L. (SIMPLIFY)

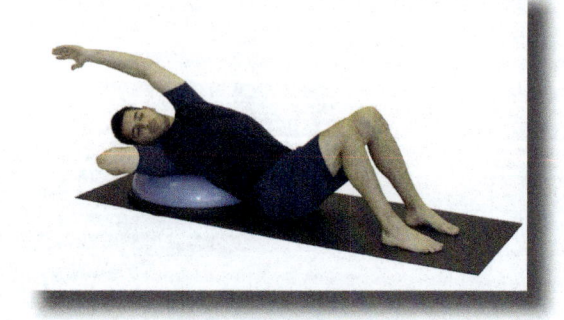

Muscular Intention

- Mobilizing the upper and middle spine.
- Opening the lateral spine (intercostals) and obliques.
- Freeing the lower spine while mobilizing the lateral flexors and extensors of the back.

Tips

- ✔ Soften the neck and shoulder muscles during the curl forward.
- ✔ Maintain the fluidity of the circle.
- ✔ Keep facing forward as you circle.
- ✔ Keep the feet and knees in line with sitting bones.
- ✔ Reach the elbows up and toward the ceiling.
- ✔ Keep the knees still.

FUNDAMENTALS

(5) TIP UPPER BODY SIDE TO SIDE

Start Position

1. Spine neutral.
2. Sitting in front of the BOSU with spine extended.
3. Hands clasped behind the head, elbows reaching toward the ceiling.
4. Knees bent slightly apart and parallel.
5. Feet on the mat and in-line with sitting bones.
6. Hips on the mat.

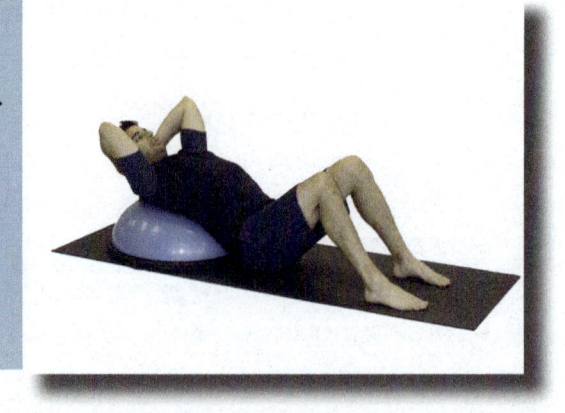

Exercise

Inhale   Tip upper body toward the R while reaching L elbow to the ceiling.

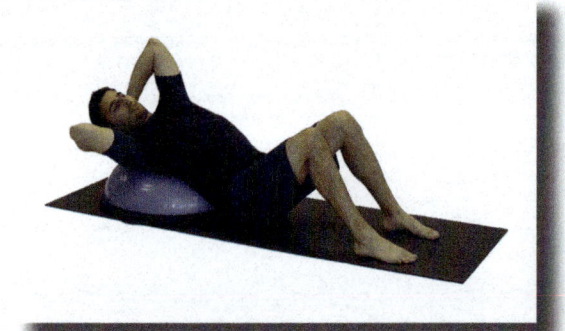

Exhale   Extend the L leg and L arm opening the L ribs, the L foot flexed.

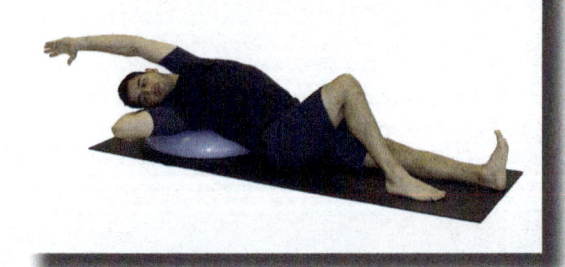

Inhale   Bend the L leg and place L hand behind the head, while reaching both elbows to the ceiling.

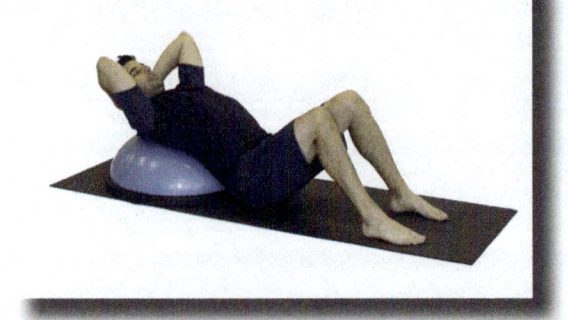

28   **EXERCISES**

Exhale	Tip upper body over to the L, extend the R leg and R arm opening the R ribs. Alternate sides
Inhale	To finish, return to **Start Position**, both hands behind head and bent knees.
Reps	X5 L/R

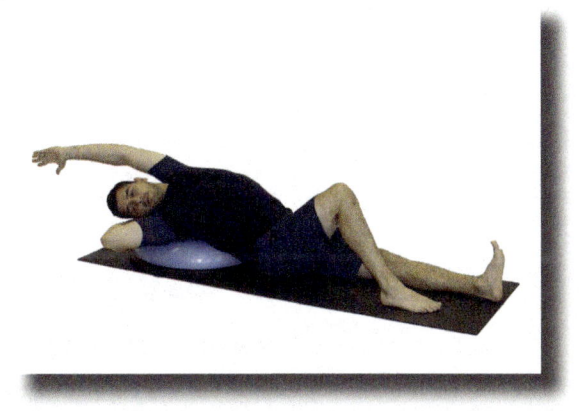

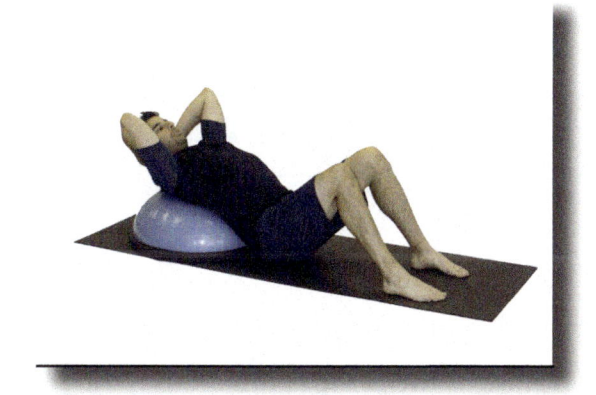

Modified

1. Tip side to side with the arm extension only, or leg extension only. Reps X5 L/R (SIMPLIFY)

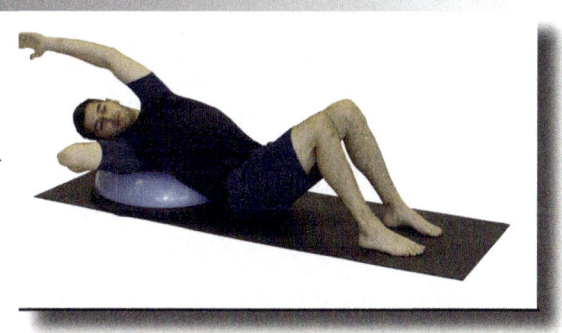

Muscular Intention

- Opening the lateral spine (intercostals) and obliques.
- Lengthening the internal abdominal obliques and hips.
- Opening the quadratus lumborum (opening between the hip bone and the bottom rib).
- Lengthening the hamstrings and the quadriceps.

Tips

- ✔ Keep the bent knee to the ceiling.
- ✔ Open the elbow you are leaning toward.
- ✔ Lengthen the hip bone away from the thigh bone.
- ✔ Support the head with the hand.
- ✔ Slide the shoulders down the back.

FUNDAMENTALS

(6) SCAPULAE ISOLATION

Start Position

1. Spine neutral.
2. Sitting on top of the dome.
3. Arms reaching overhead to ceiling.
4. Palms face each other.
5. Knees bent slightly apart and parallel.
6. Feet on the mat and in-line with sitting bones.

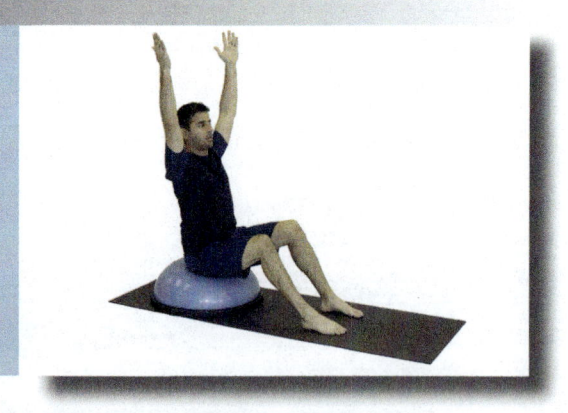

Exercise

Inhale   Shrug the shoulders up to the ears.
              Palms face away from one another.

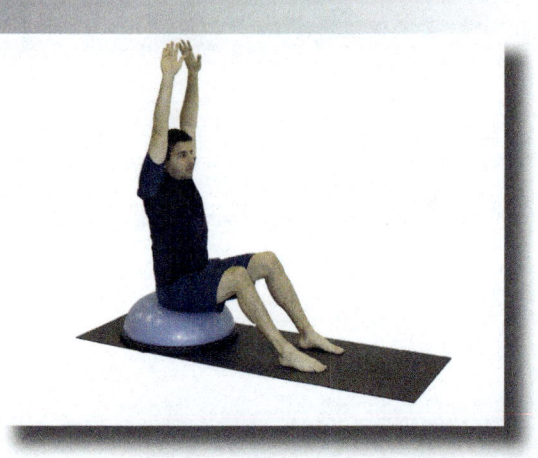

Exhale   Slide the shoulders down the back.
              Palms face one another.

Reps   X5-10

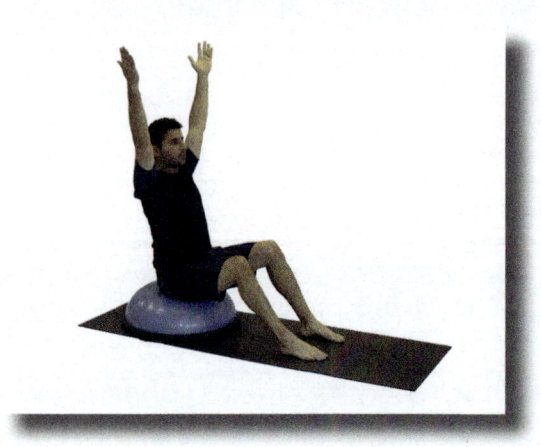

Modified

1. Elevate and depress the shoulder blades. Arms reaching forward to shoulder height. Lift the shoulders up to your ears, then slide the shoulders down the back. Reps X5-10 (SIMPLIFY)

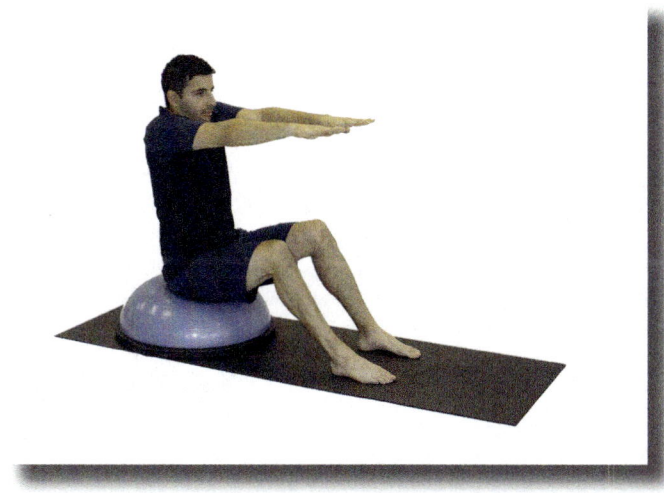

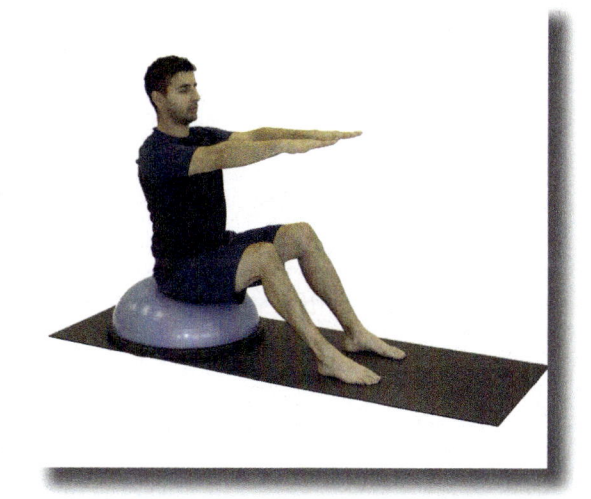

2. Protract and retract. Reach the arms forward to open the upper back then slide the shoulders down the back, spine to neutral. Reps X5-10 (SIMPLIFY)

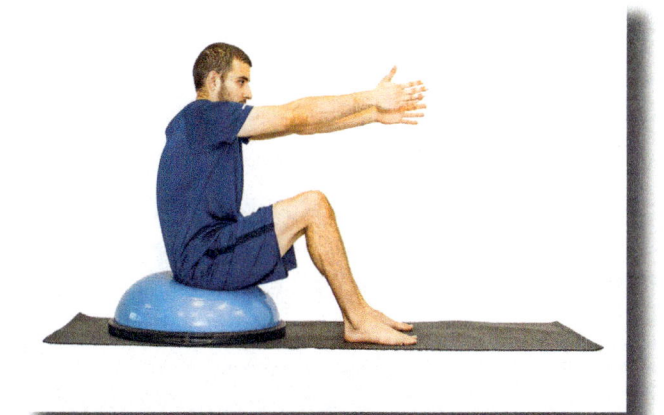

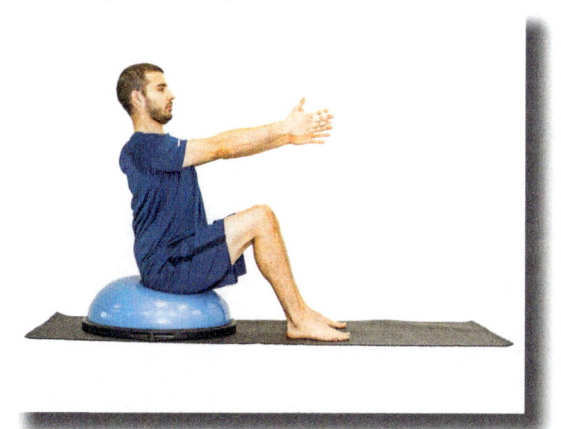

Muscular Intention

- Stabilizing latissimus dorsi, rhomboids, and teres major.
- Increasing the length in the cervical spine.

Tips

✔ Slide the shoulders down the back and keep the collar bones open.
✔ Maintain neutral pelvis and sit on top of the sitting bones.
✔ Keep the knees and feet parallel.
✔ Push both feet into the mat to increase the length of the spine.

FUNDAMENTALS

(7) ARM CIRCLES

Start Position

1. Spine neutral.
2. Head and shoulders on the top of the dome.
3. Chest and ribs against the front half of the dome.
4. Arms reaching toward feet, palms face each other.
5. Knees bent slightly apart and parallel.
6. Feet on the mat and in-line with sitting bones.
7. Hips on the mat.

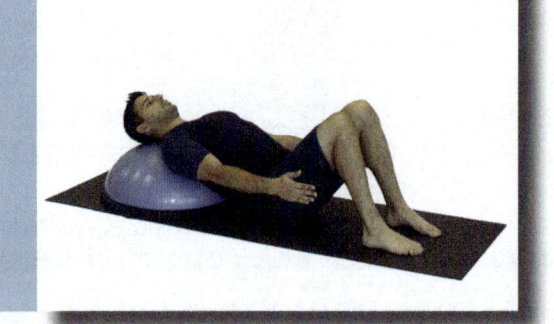

Exercise

Inhale   Reach the arms overhead, palms face each other.

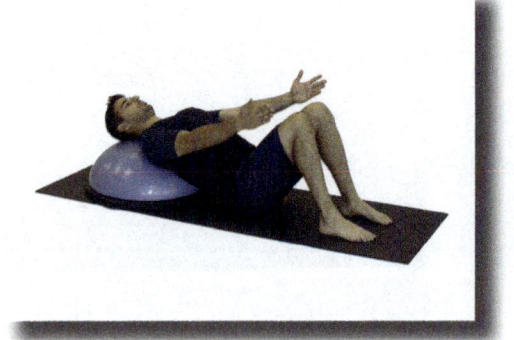

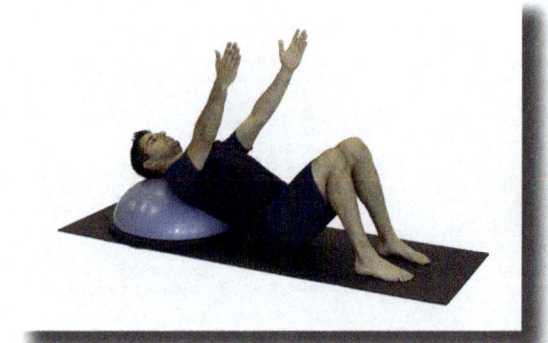

Exhale   Circle the arms out to the sides, and down toward the calves.

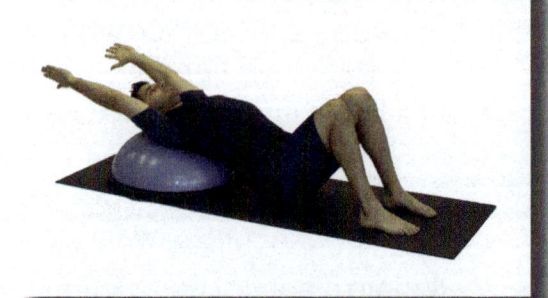

Reach your arms to your ears.

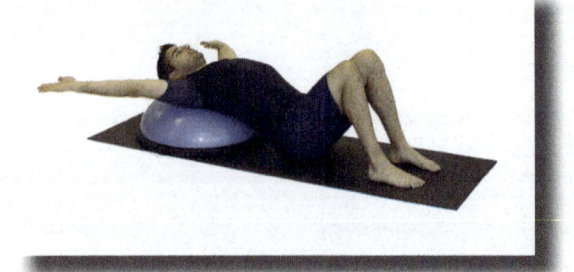

Open arms to a V.

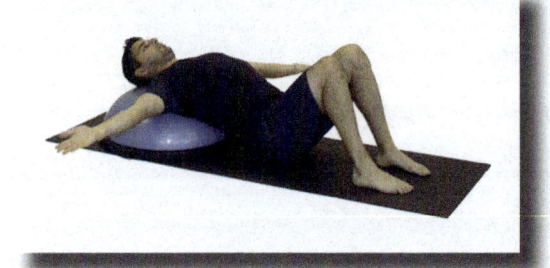

Continue circle down toward heels.

32   EXERCISES

Inhale   Return to **Start Position**, palms face down or face each other.

Reps   X5-10

» Repeat in reverse.

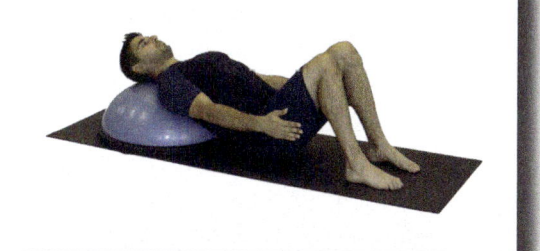

Modified

1. Lift the arms overhead, then lower the arms straight down. Reps X5 (SIMPLIFY)

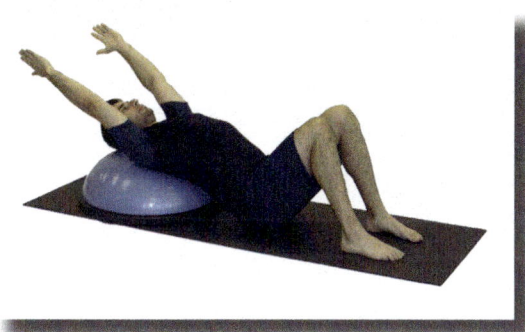

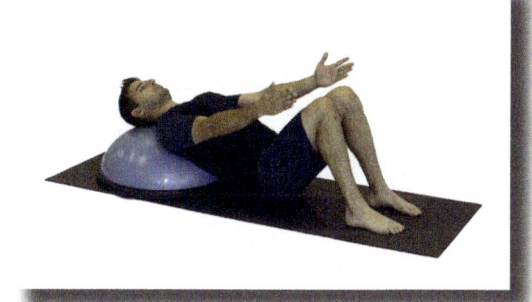

2. Palms out to the sides then down - imagine, jumping jack arms. Reps X10 (SIMPLIFY)

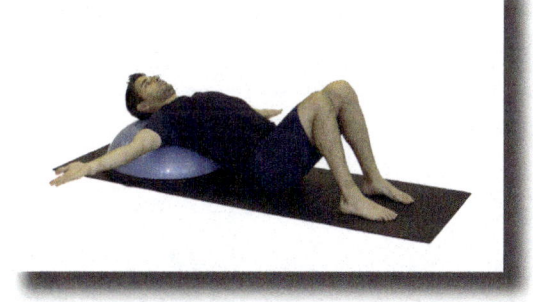

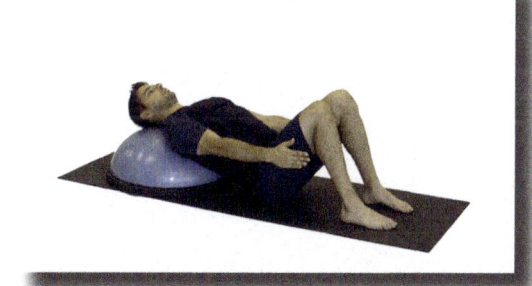

Muscular Intention

- Stabilizing latissimus dorsi, rhomboids, and teres major.
- Opening the pectorals and sternum.
- Releasing tension in your upper trapezius.
- Lengthening the cervical spine.

Tips

✔ Keep arms fluid during circles.
✔ Slide the shoulders down the back and keep the collar bones wide.
✔ Connect the bottom ribs to the hip bones.
✔ Maintain neutral pelvis.
✔ If the head on top of the dome puts a strain on the neck, place a pillow or towel under the head or slide down so the neck is more comfortable.

FUNDAMENTALS

(8) ABDOMINALS

Start Position

1. Spine neutral.
2. Sit in front of the BOSU, lower back against the front half of the dome.
3. Extend the upper body backwards over the top of the dome.
4. Hands clasped behind the head.
5. Elbows angling out from the ears, and forward.
6. Knees bent slightly apart and parallel.
7. Feet on the mat and in-line with sitting bones.

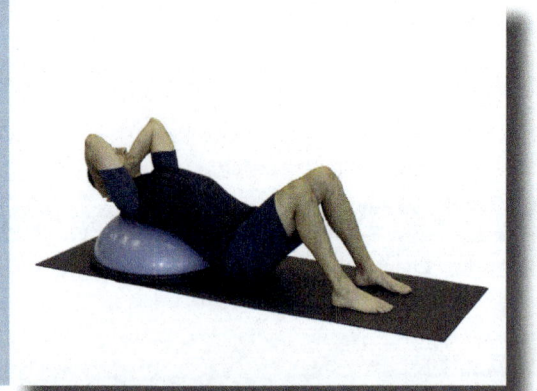

Exercise

Inhale Lengthen the spine into extension and prepare.

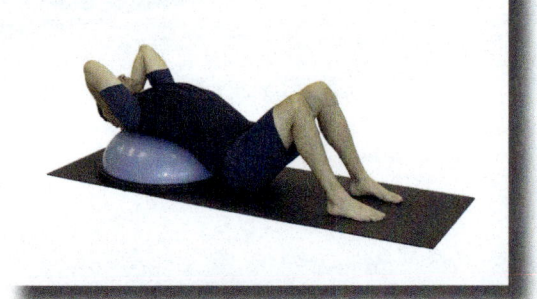

Exhale Curl upper body forward, sliding the rib cage toward the hips, pelvis imprinted.

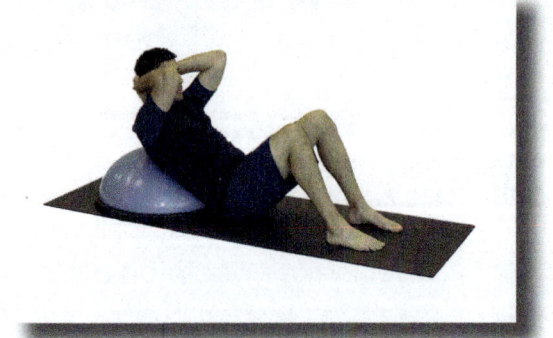

Inhale Hold and increase spinal flexion.

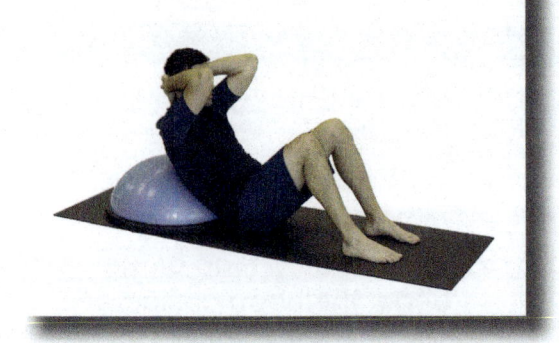

Exhale   Lengthen and extend the spine back to **Start Position**.
Reps   X5-10

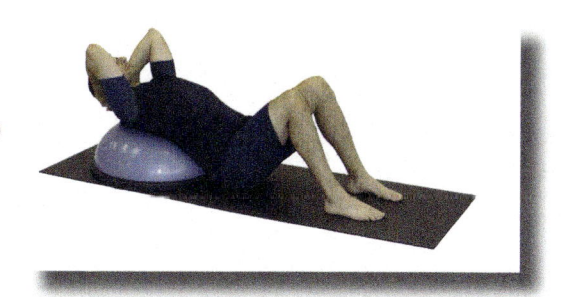

Modified

1. Head and shoulders against the dome, low spine along mat, arms reaching. Reps X5 (ASSIST)

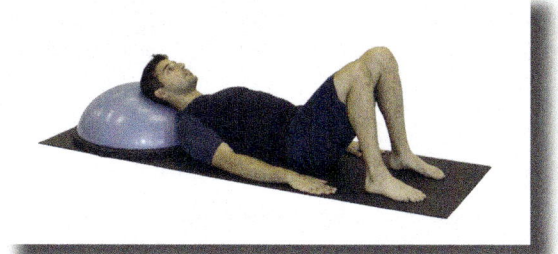

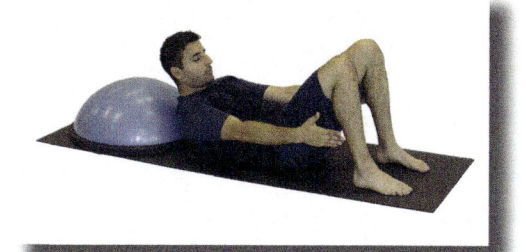

2. Head, shoulders and spine on mat, legs over the top of dome. Reps X5 (CHALLENGE)

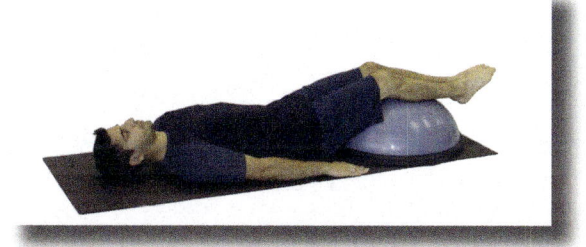

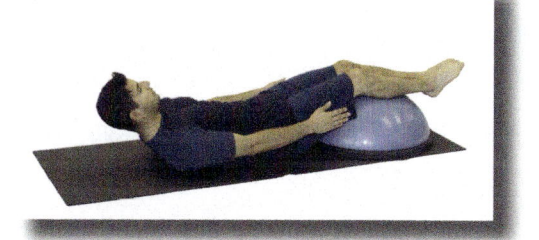

3. Feet on the dome, together or slightly apart. With hands behind the head. Reps X10 (ASSIST)

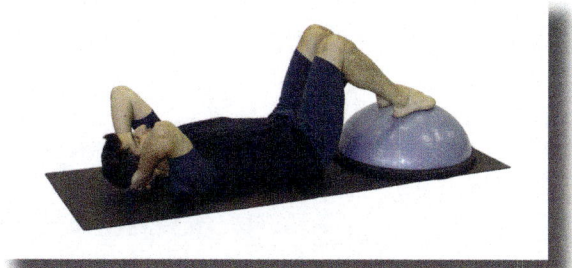

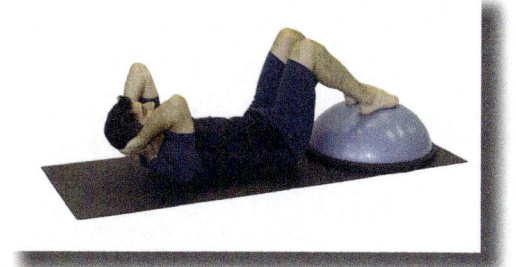

Muscular Intention

- Stabilizing and flexing the spine using abdominals.
- Maintaining scapular depression using scapular stabilizers.
- Stabilizing pelvis in neutral using transverse abdominus and internal abdominal obliques.

Tips

✔ Feet in line with sitting bones.
✔ Slide the shoulders down the back and keep the collar bones wide.

FUNDAMENTALS

(9) BREAST STROKE PREP

Start Position

1. Prone.
2. Low spine neutral with belly on top of the bull's eye.
3. Upper spine is softly curled forward.
4. Forearms parallel on the mat with palms down.
5. Head soft between arms, neck and chest forward.
6. Legs are slightly apart and relaxed, knees are bent.
7. Feet pointed.

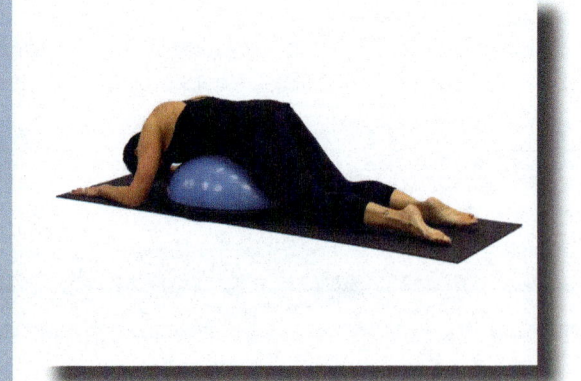

Exercise

Inhale	Engage low **abdominals**, sliding shoulders down the back and simultaneously lift the head and chest to neutral and flex the feet.
Exhale	Extend the arms and upper spine, lifting head and chest (long neck).
Inhale	Hold position and lengthen the spine.
Exhale	Return to **Start Position**.
Reps	X5-10

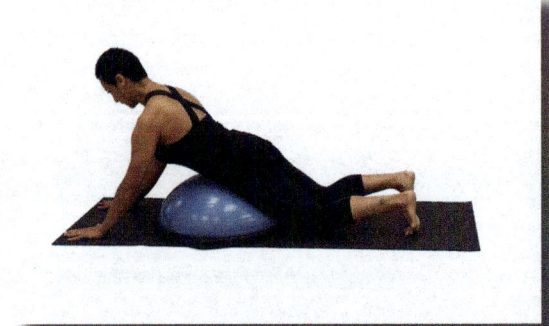

36 EXERCISES

Modified

1. Upper body hover above the mat, hands beside the thighs hugging the dome, knees on the mat. Extend and flex upper spine. Reps X5-10 (SIMPLIFY)

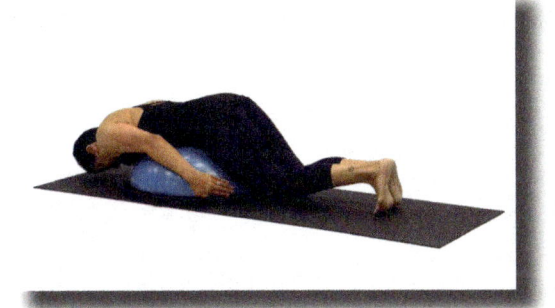

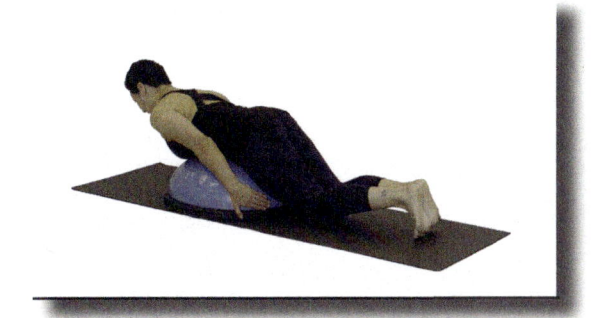

2. Torpedo prep. Straighten the knees, feet are flexed on the mat. Hands on the dome next to thighs. Extend and lift both legs off the mat, pointing both feet, keeping knees straight. Simultaneously bringing both hands to the thighs. Reps X5-10 (CHALLENGE)

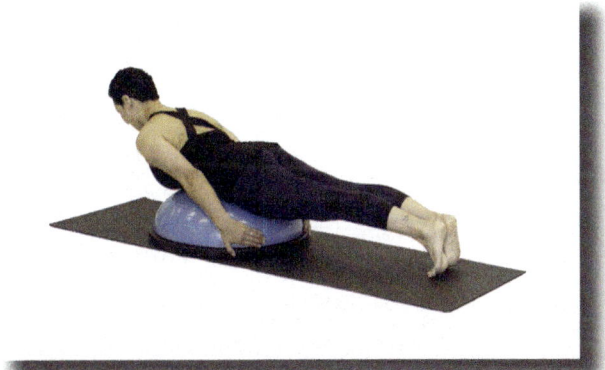

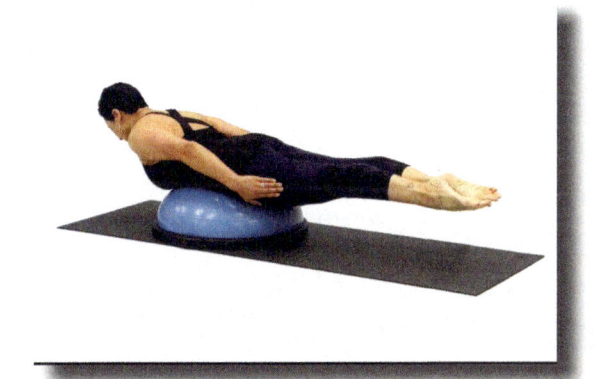

Muscular Intention

- Emphasizing mid-thoracic spine during extension.
- Lengthening and strengthening of the latissimus dorsi and paraspinals.
- Maintaining scapular depression using scapular stabilizers.
- Supporting spine using abdominals.
- Straightening the legs using glutes and hamstrings.

Tips

✔ Engage the abdominals throughout.
✔ Lengthen the head away from the heels.
✔ Slide the shoulders down the back and keep the collar bones wide.

FUNDAMENTALS

(10) CHILD'S POSE

Start Position

1. Knees on the dome with buttocks hovering above the heels.
2. Feet and knees together.
3. Spine in C curve.
4. Arms extended, with fingers spread on the mat.
5. Head between the arms.
6. Toes on the mat, tucked under.

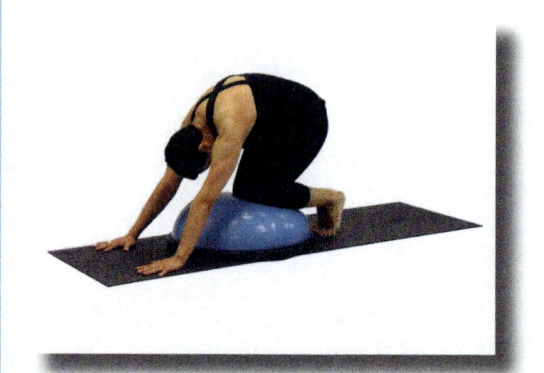

Exercise

Inhale   Deepen the C curve.
Exhale   Place the emphasis on the lower back to increase flexion, curving from the tailbone to the top of the head.
Reps   X5 Breaths

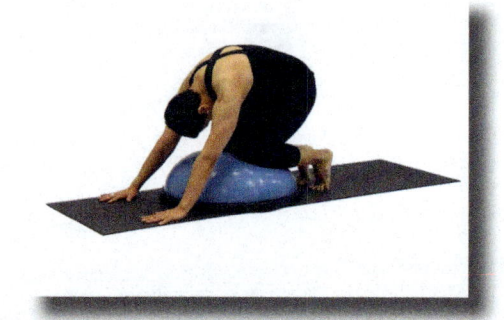

Modified

1. Rocking Child's Pose: Glutes on/off heels. Push into both hands to stretch the back. Ankles and knees together or slightly apart. Reps X5 Breaths (SIMPLIFY)

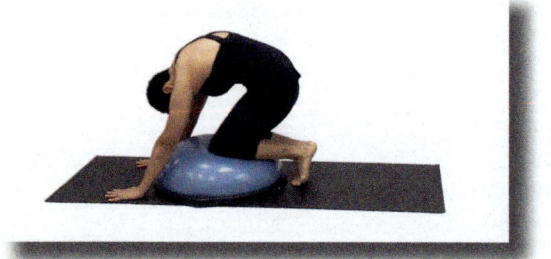

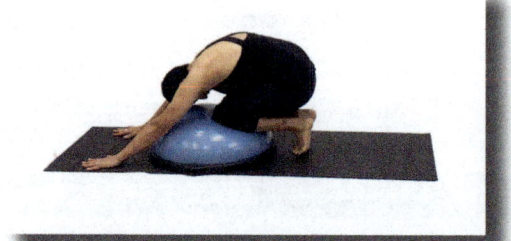

2. Shins on the mat. Hands on the dome. Aim to keep inner thighs and heels together.
Reps X5 Breaths (SIMPLIFY)

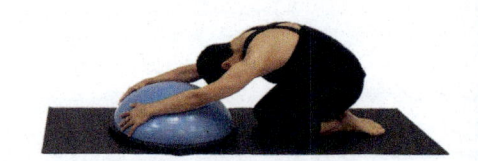

38   EXERCISES

3. Shins on the dome. Knees and ankles together. Push hands into the mat. Reps X5 Breaths (CHALLENGE)

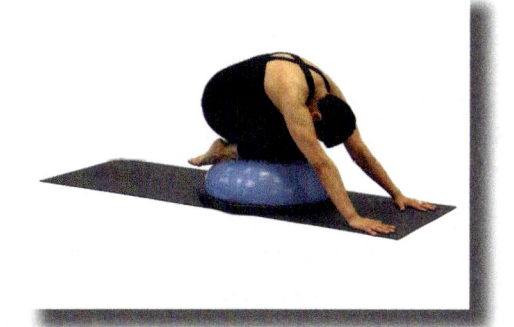

Muscular Intention

- Stretching back extensors.
- Keeping the knees and feet together using the adductors.
- Increasing the flexibility of both wrists by spreading fingers.

Tips

- ✔ Massage the lower back using abdominals.
- ✔ Open the thoracic spine by pushing both hands into the mat.
- ✔ Press the knees and shins into the dome.
- ✔ Push into the palms while spreading the fingers wide.

(11) HUNDRED

Start Position

1. Spine neutral.
2. Head and shoulders on top of the dome.
3. Arms reaching toward feet, elbows are soft, palms down.
4. Hips and feet on the mat.
5. Knees bent slightly apart and parallel.
6. Feet on the mat and in-line with sitting bones.

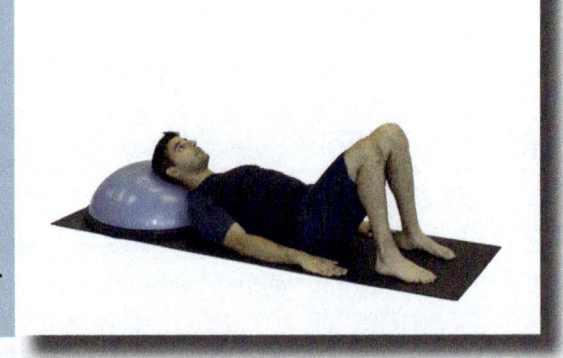

Exercise

Inhale   Lengthen spine and hover the arms above the mat.

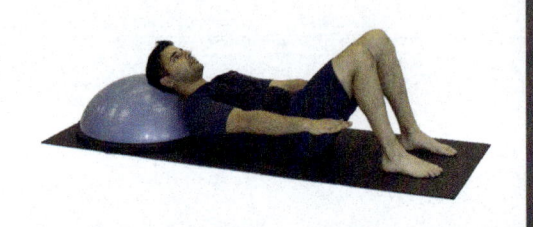

Exhale   Curl the upper body forward, reaching the arms toward the feet.

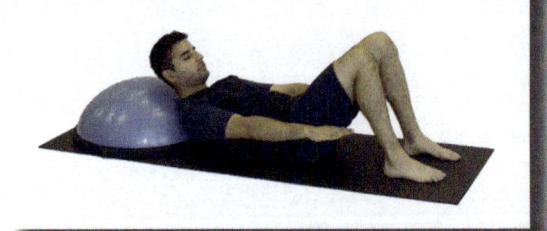

Inhale   ...2345 breaths – Pulse arms up and down.

Exhale   ...2345 breaths – Pulse arms up and down (this is one cycle).

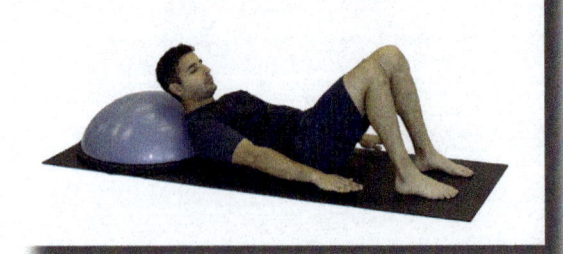

40   **EXERCISES**

To Finish...

Inhale   Remain in curl, reaching arms even more.

Exhale   Return the head and shoulders back to **Start Position**.

Reps   X10 Cycles

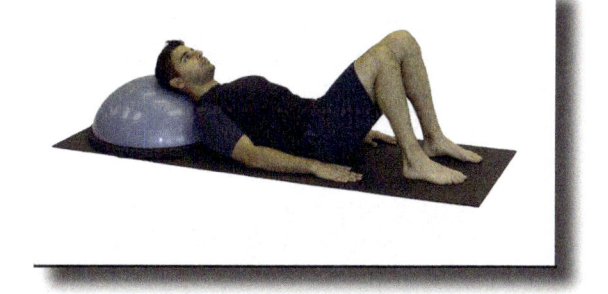

Modified

1. Head and shoulders on the mat and hips on the dome (legs to table top, hands hold the dome). Practice the breathing only.
Reps X10 Cycles (ASSIST)

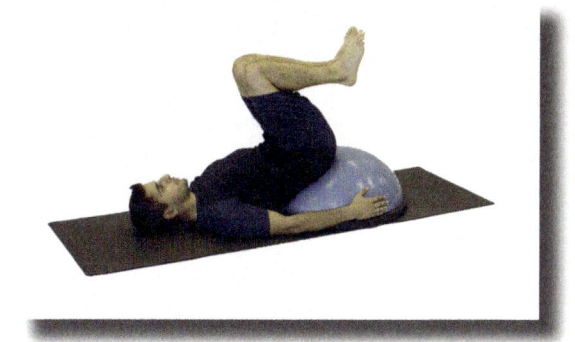

2. Head forward or on the dome. Shoulders supported on the dome, buttocks off the mat. Bridge position. Place one hand behind head. (Breathing only). Reps X10 Cycles (SIMPLIFY)

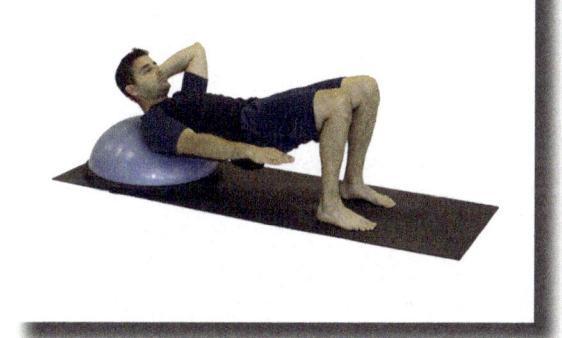

3. Flat side up. Curl forward and place one hand behind the head. Pulse the single arm. Reps X10 Cycles (CHALLENGE)

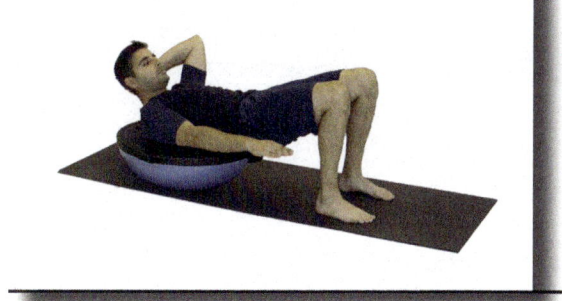

FUNDAMENTALS

Muscular Intention

- Engaging the abdominals through the action of the breath.
- Stabilize and flex the spine using abdominals and glutes.
- Supporting the arms using the scapular stabilizers.

Tips

- ✔ Slide the shoulders down the back and keep the collar bones wide.
- ✔ Deepen the abdominal connection throughout.
- ✔ Reach the elbow toward the ceiling when using one hand behind the head.
- ✔ Maintain correct breathing rhythms.
- ✔ Keep the dome level on the flat side.
- ✔ Push into both feet to lift hips.

(12) HALF ROLL BACK

Start Position

1. Spine lengthened, and pelvis neutral.
2. Place sitting bones slightly in front of bulls eye on dome.
3. Arms reaching forward at shoulder height. Palms face down.
4. Knees bent slightly apart and parallel.
5. Feet on the mat and in-line with sitting bones.

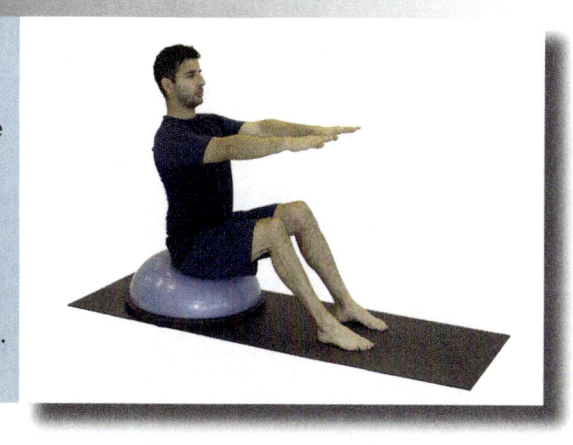

Exercise

Inhale	Lengthen the spine by pushing both feet into the floor.
Exhale	Engage the lower glutes and abdominals and roll back off the sitting bones into posterior pelvic tilt.
Inhale	Hold the lumbar curve.
Exhale	Return back onto the sitting bones and extend spine to **Start Position**.
Reps	X5

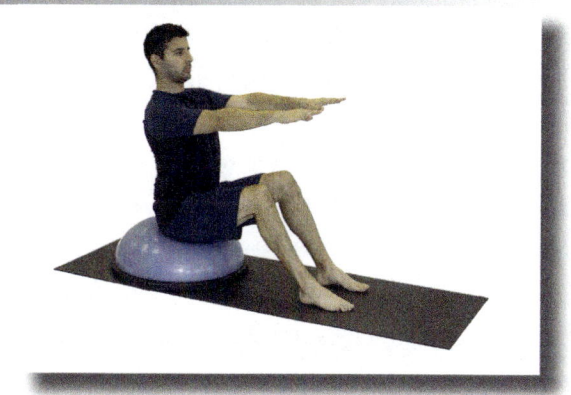

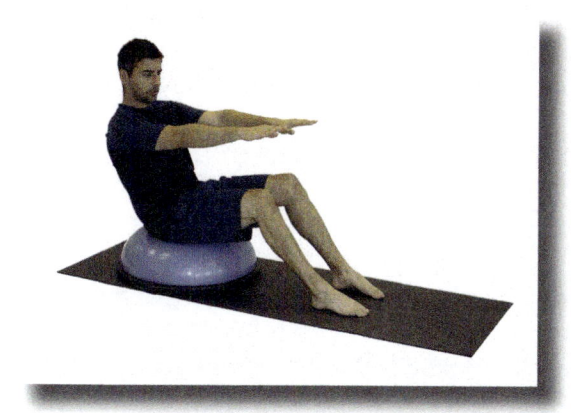

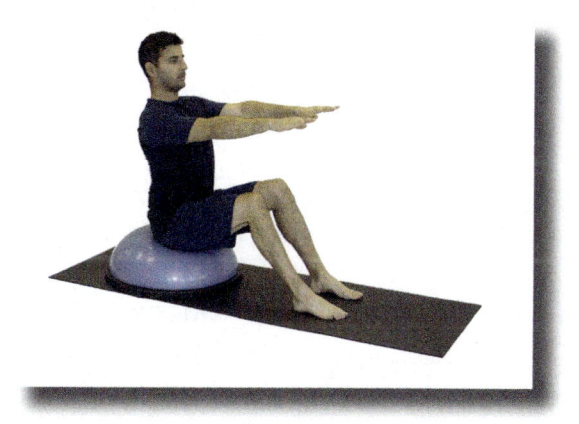

FUNDAMENTALS 43

Modified

1. Sit slightly away from BOSU on the mat. Knees bent with legs slightly apart, hands behind the knees. Reps X5 (ASSIST)

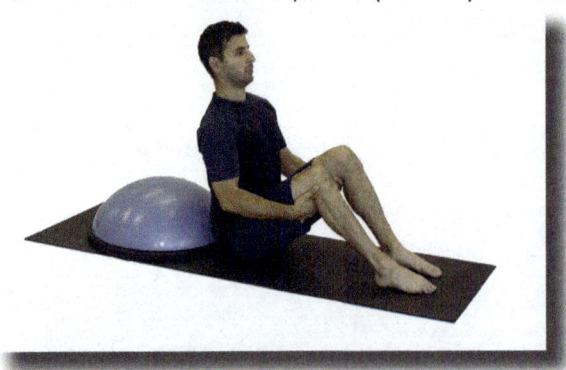

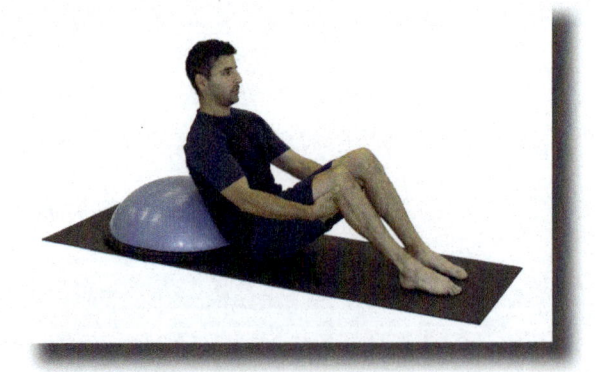

2. Hold the C-curve on top of the dome and lift one leg at a time. Reps X5 (CHALLENGE)

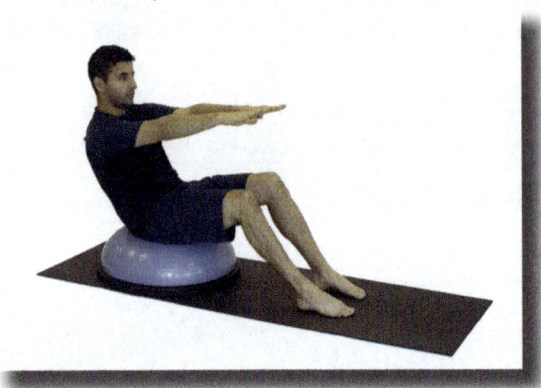

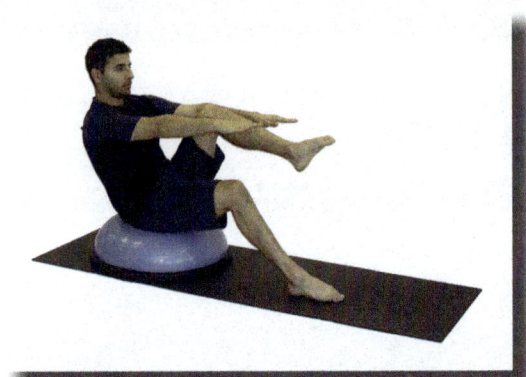

3. Elevate one leg at a time with hands behind knees. Reps X5 (CHALLENGE)

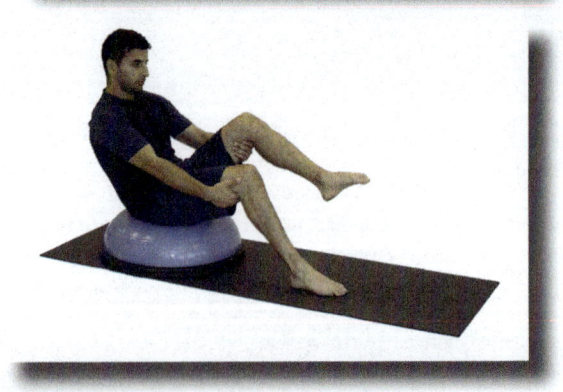

Muscular Intention

- Abdominals and hip flexors concentrically contract on roll back and eccentrically contract on return.
- Maintaining scapular depression using scapular stabilizers.
- Engaging hamstrings and lower glutes.
- Working the deep transverse abdominus and internal abdominal obliques.

Tips

✔ Slide the shoulders down the back and keep the collar bones wide.
✔ Increase the connection of the lower abdominals.
✔ Push both feet into floor to engage the hamstrings and lower glutes during the half rollback.

(13) ROLL UP PREP

Start Position

1. Sitting in front of the BOSU on the mat.
2. Head and shoulders resting on the dome. If neck tension, place a pillow or towel under the head or slide down so the neck is more comfortable.
3. Spine extended back over the dome.
4. Arms reach overhead, soft elbows.
5. Knees bent slightly apart and parallel.
6. Feet on the mat and in-line with sitting bones.

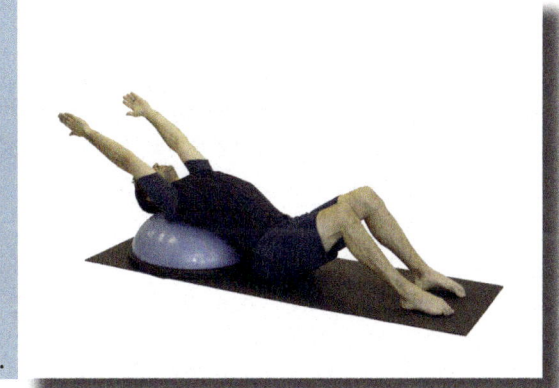

Exercise

Inhale — Lift arms to ceiling.

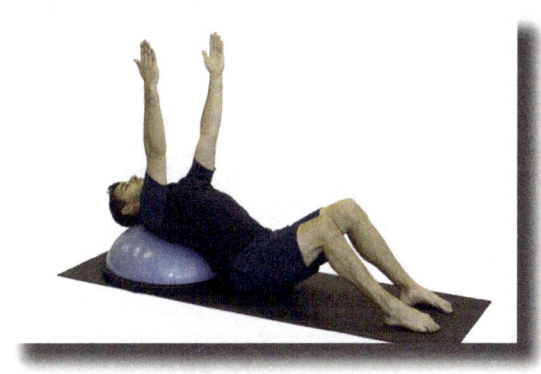

Exhale — Curl upper body forward reaching arms toward knees. Straighten your legs as you continue to curl forward.

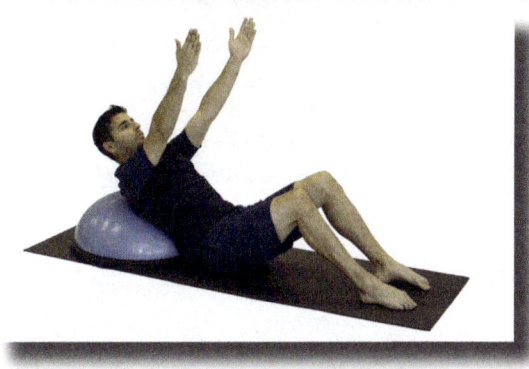

Start to curl forward reaching both arms to the ceiling.

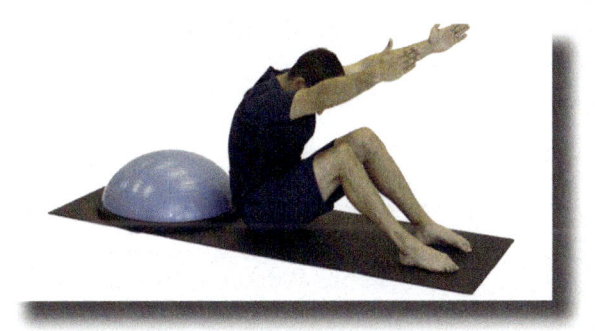

Deepen the curl. Roll away from the dome.

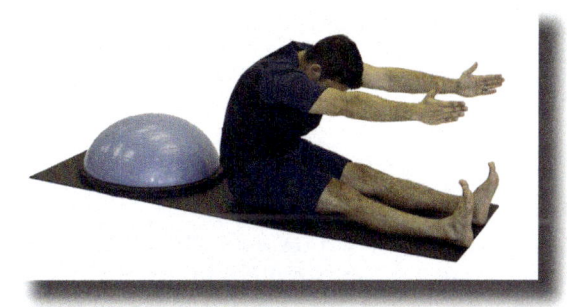

Straighten the legs, reaching the head between the legs.

FUNDAMENTALS 45

Inhale   Reach the head between the arms, increase the lower curve, touching the lower spine to the dome.

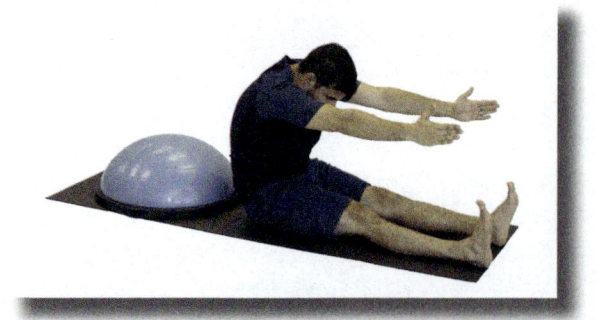

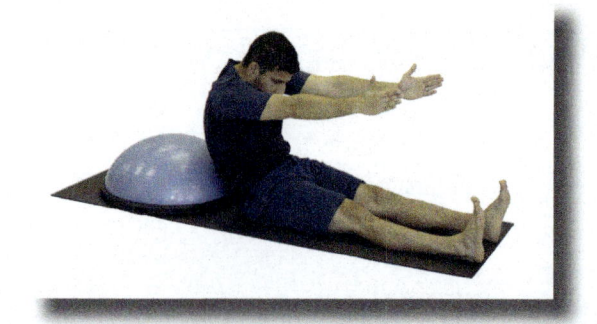

Exhale   Roll back into the dome, bend the knees and send arms back overhead to **Start Position.**

Reps   X5-10

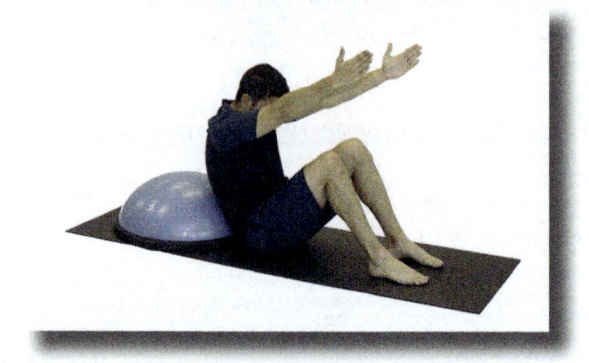

Modified

1. Place hands behind the head, low back against the dome with straight legs. Flex and extend the upper body only. Reps X5-10 (ASSIST)

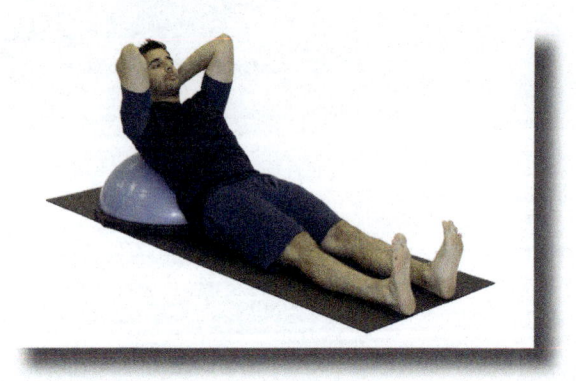

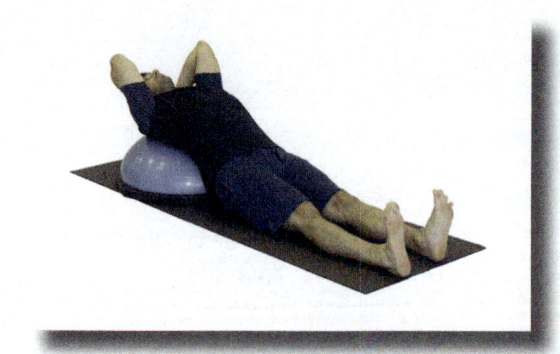

2. Legs can stay bent throughout the roll-ups. Reps X5-10 (SIMPLIFY)

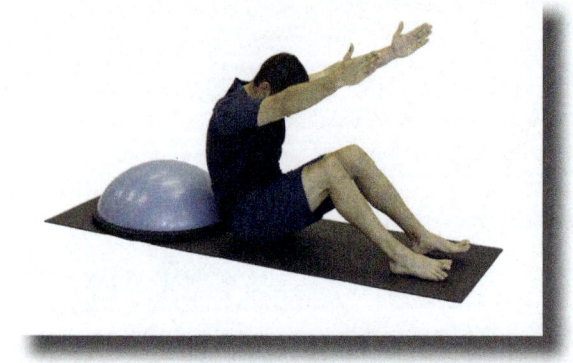

EXERCISES

Muscular Intention

- Stabilizing the spine using transverse abdominus
- Flexing the spine using rectus abdominus and internal abdominal obliques.
- Maintaining scapular depression using scapular stabilizers.
- Straightening the legs using glutes and hamstrings.

Tips

- ✔ Slide the shoulders down the back and keep the collar bones wide.
- ✔ Articulate each vertebra one at a time as you roll away and toward the dome.
- ✔ Breath into the back before rolling back onto the dome.

(14) SINGLE LEG CIRCLE

Start Position

1. Spine is imprinted.
2. Sitting with spine scooped in front of the BOSU on the mat.
3. Place hands behind the head.
4. R leg bent with foot pointed in tabletop.
5. L foot on the mat.

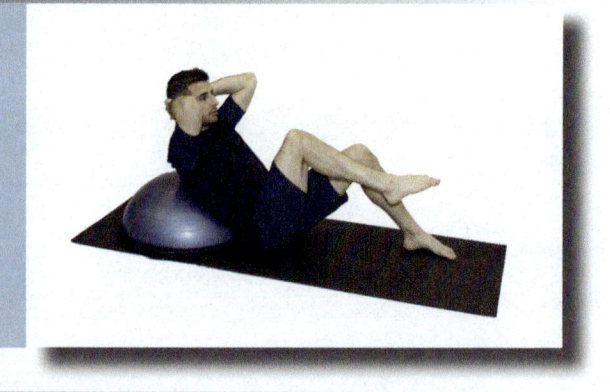

Exercise

Inhale   Circling R leg CCW to 12 o'clock (think about circling from the knee, not the foot).

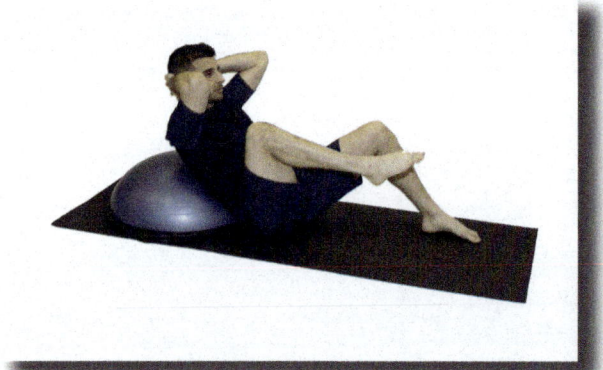

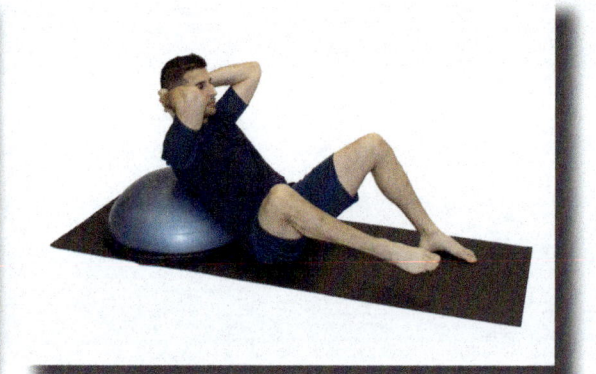

Exhale   Circling R leg CCW to 6 o'clock.
Reps   X5

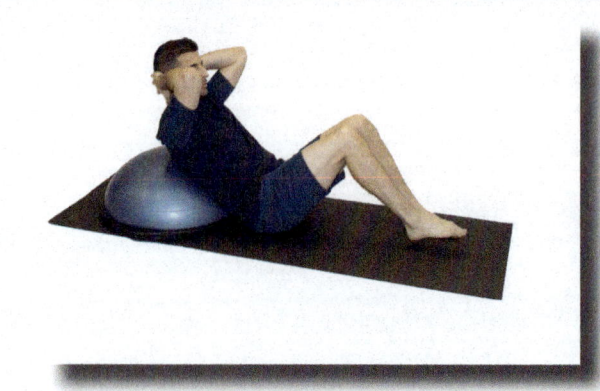

Reverse...
Inhale   Circling R leg CW to 12 o'clock.
Exhale   Circling R leg CW to 6 o'clock.
Reps   X5

Inhale   Return R leg to mat.

» Repeat on L leg.

Modified

1. Press both hands into the mat beside hips and connect deeper into the abdominals. Reps X5 L/R (ASSIST)

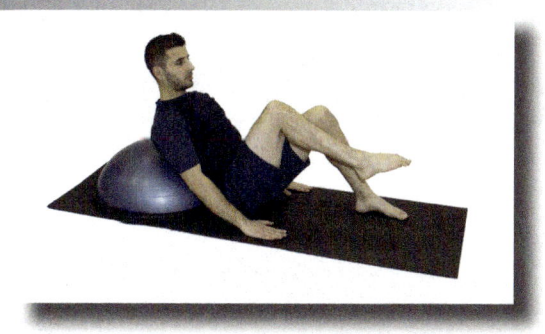

2. Head and shoulders on the mat, hips on the dome one foot on the mat, the other leg bent (option a) or extended to the ceiling (option b). Reps X5 L/R (CHALLENGE)

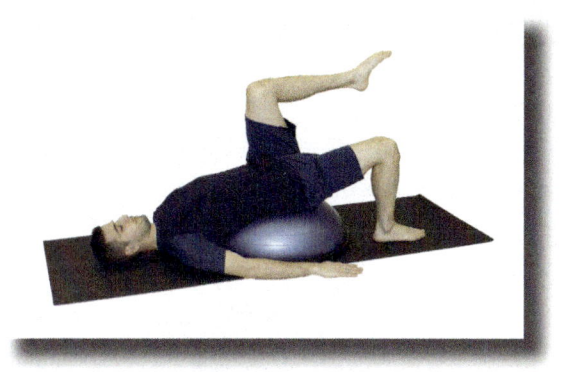

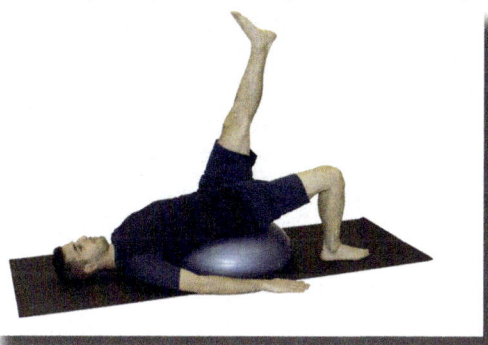

option a   option b

3. Lift hips a little higher with hands behind the head. Reps X5 L/R (CHALLENGE)

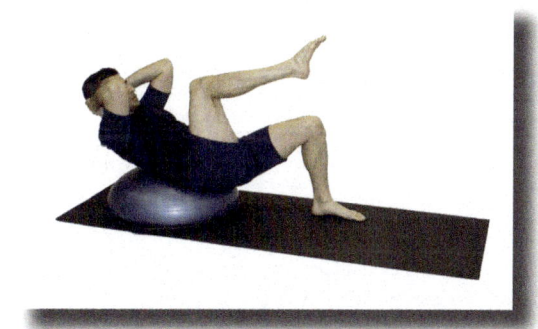

Muscular Intention
- Stabilizing pelvis using abdominals, specifically obliques during circles.
- Co-ordinating circumduction action of the hip flexors and hamstrings using adductors and abductors.
- Stabilizing the hamstrings, glutes and obliques while pushing the supporting foot into the mat.

Tips
- ✔ Slide the shoulders down the back and keep the collar bones wide.
- ✔ Deepen the abdominal connection.
- ✔ Control the leg circle by pushing down into the supporting foot.
- ✔ Keep the supporting knee and foot parallel to the ceiling.
- ✔ Initiate the circle from the bent knee and not the foot.

FUNDAMENTALS

(15) SITTING SPINE TWIST

Start Position

1. Sit on top of the dome.
2. Spine is neutral.
3. Arms extended to the sides at shoulder height, palms facing mat.
4. Knees bent slightly apart and parallel.
5. Feet on the mat and in-line with sitting bones.

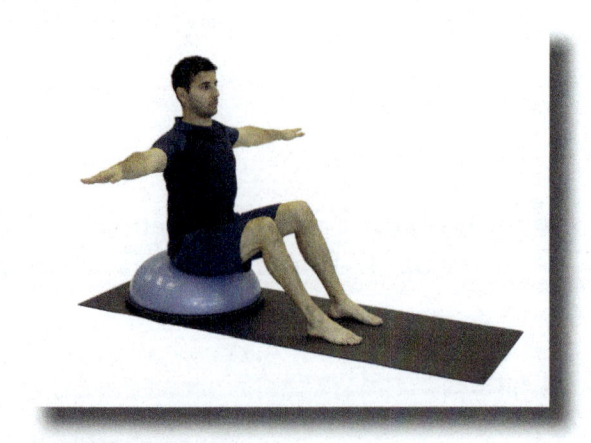

Exercise

Inhale   3 inhalations rotating R and lengthening the spine (corner, side wall, look back over the R arm).

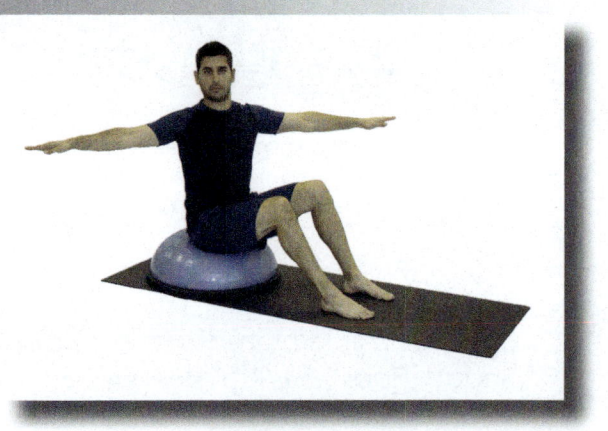

Rotate to the front L corner

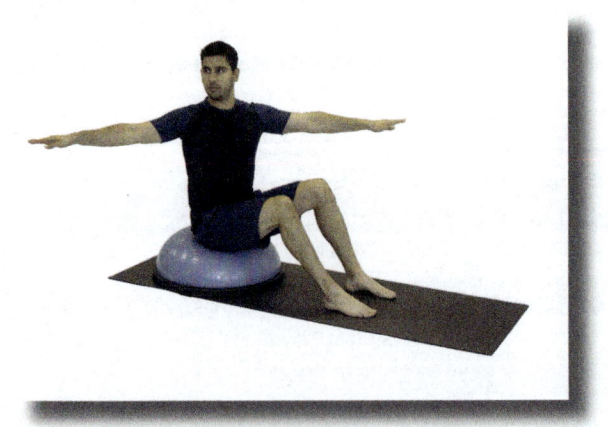

Increase rotation to the side

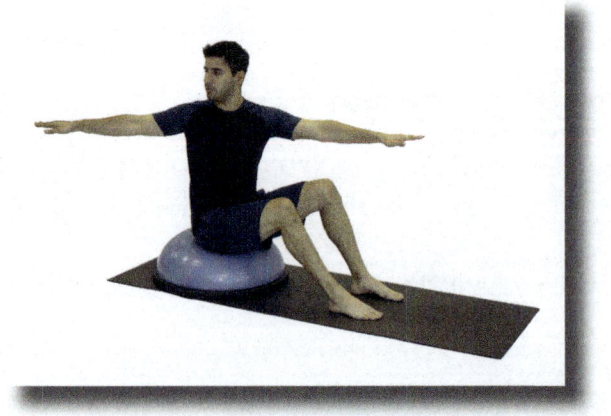

Increase rotation to the back wall

50 **EXERCISES**

Inhale   Repeat rotation to L.
Exhale   Return to **Start Position**.
Reps   X5 L/R

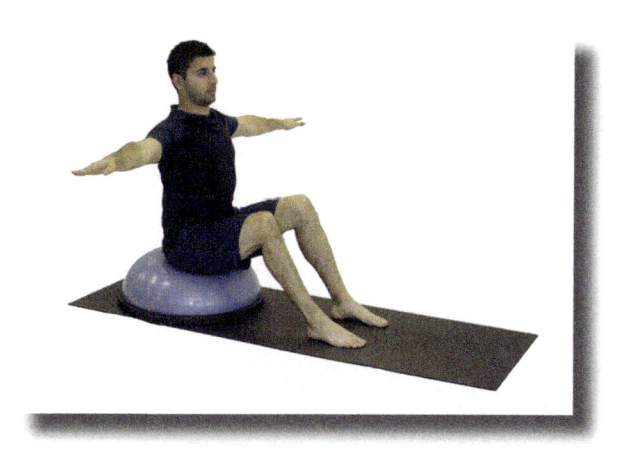

Exhale   Return to **Start Position**.

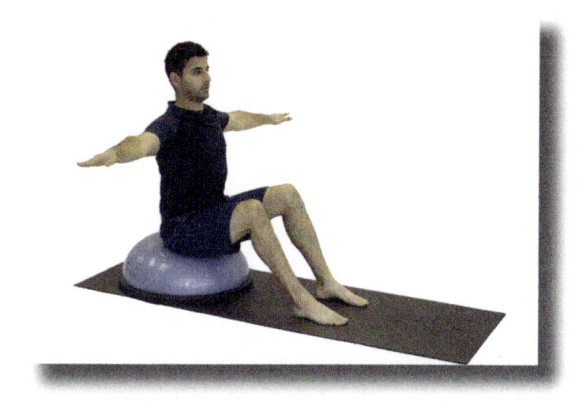

Modified

1. Hold hands to elbows, knees and feet parallel. Reps X3-5 L/R (SIMPLIFY)
2. Reverse breathing. Reps X3-5 L/R (CHALLENGE)

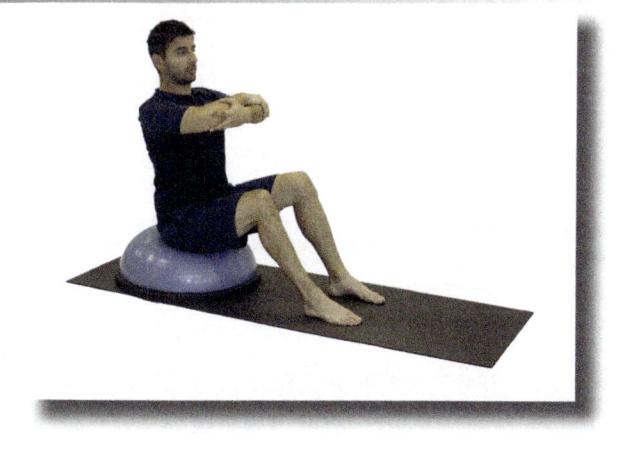

3. One arm bent, the other straight. Reps X3-5 L/R (CHALLENGE)

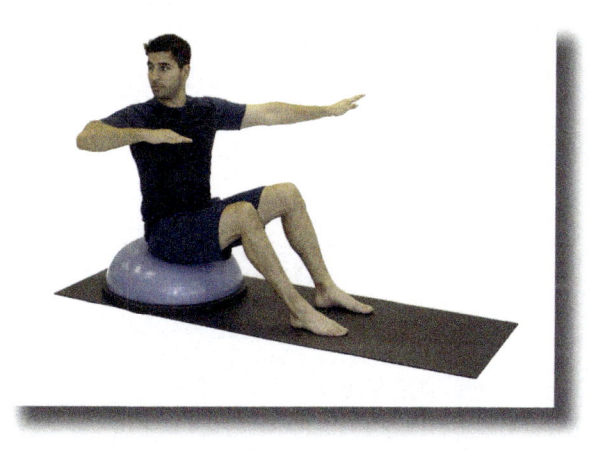

FUNDAMENTALS   51

4. Cross one leg over the other. Twist the spine to the L side and then the R side, then change the legs. Reps X3-5 L/R (CHALLENGE)

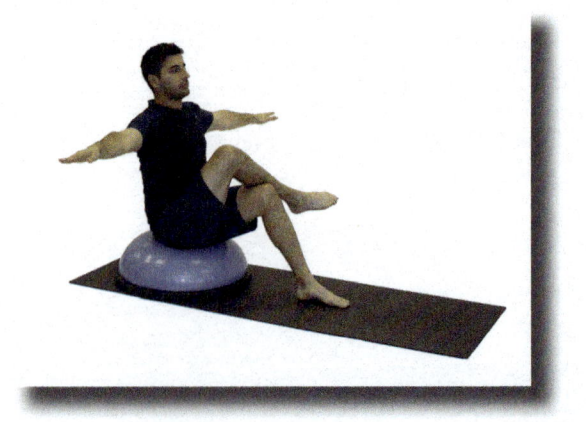

5. Flat side up. Reps X3-5 L/R (CHALLENGE)

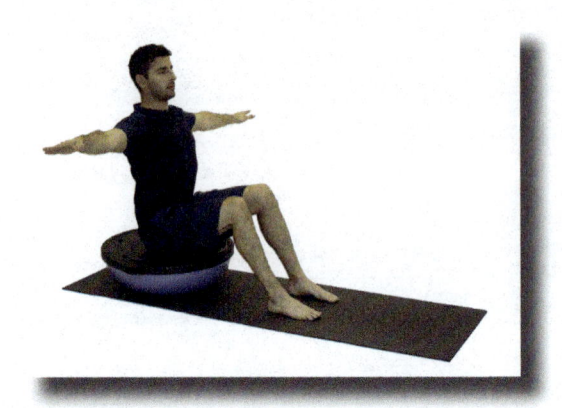

Muscular Intention
- Stabilizing the arms using **latissimus dorsi, rhomboids**, and **teres major**.
- Increasing the length in the **cervical spine** using the deep paraspinals.
- Rotating the **spine** using **obliques** and **paraspinals**.
- Maintaining scapular depression using **scapular stabilizers**.

Tips
- ✔ Maintain neutral **pelvis** throughout the twist.
- ✔ Deepen the **abdominal connection**
- ✔ Slide the shoulders down the back and keep the **collar bones** wide.
- ✔ Increase the length of the **spine** as you rotate.

52   EXERCISES

(16) SIDE LYING LATERAL OBLIQUES

Start Position

1. Lying on R side with torso and hips on the dome.
2. R elbow and forearm on the mat, hand in a fist.
3. Head in line with the spine, looking straight ahead or down to the R elbow.
4. Reach L arm overhead.
5. Spine and pelvis neutral with hips stacked.
6. Both legs together and extended with feet flexed.

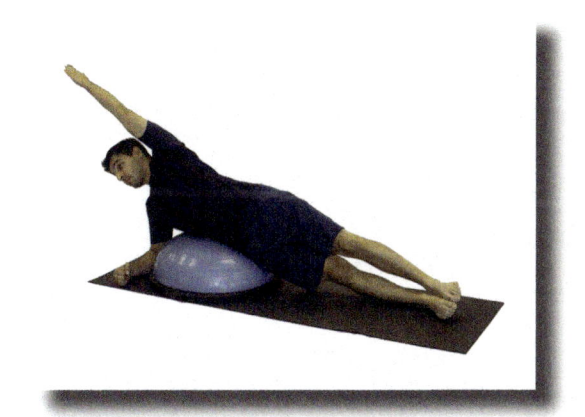

Exercise

Inhale   Increase reaching the L arm away from left leg.

Exhale   Flex the L elbow to L knee, turned out. Keep the hips stacked.

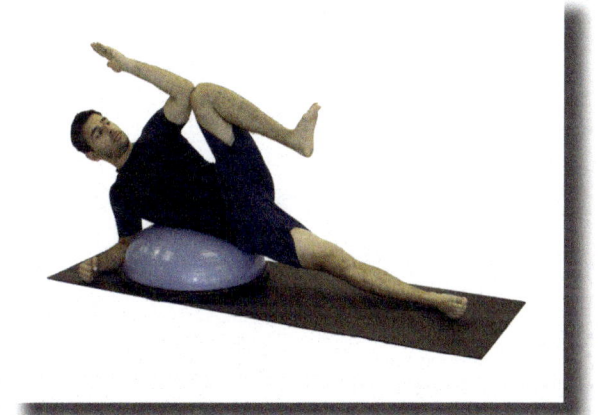

Inhale   To extend to **Start Position.**
Reps   X10

» Repeat on L side.

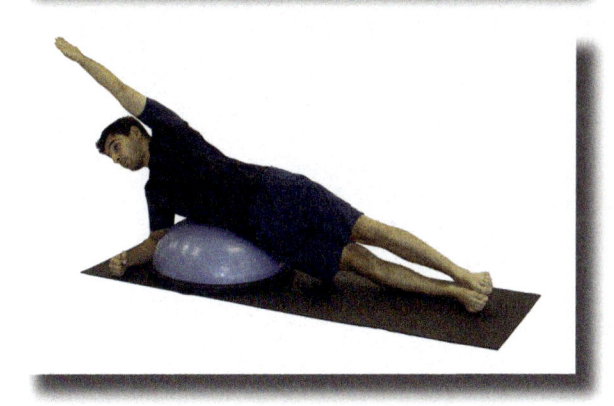

FUNDAMENTALS   53

Modified

1. Hips on the mat. R hand supports the head. Bottom knee bent. Bring L elbow to L knee, L leg turned out. Reps X10 L/R (CHALLENGE)

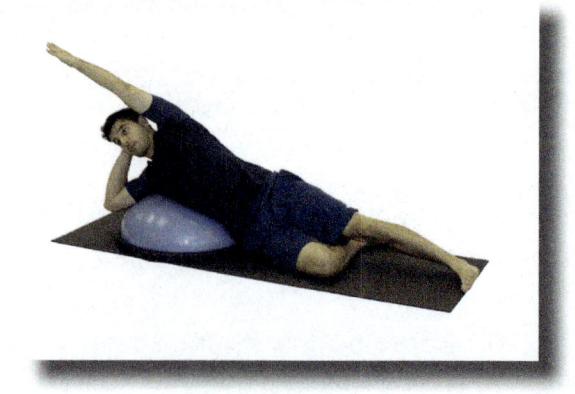

2. Bring the hips higher on top of the dome. Forearm on the mat. Bottom knee bent. Bring L elbow to L knee, L leg turned out. Reps X10 L/R (CHALLENGE)

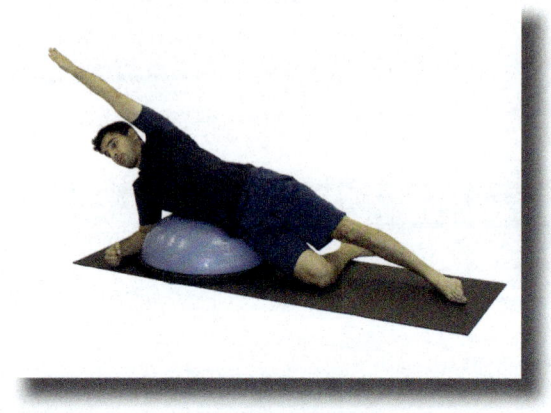

Muscular Intention
- Stabilizing hips using abdominals especially the internal abdominal obliques.
- Strengthening the flexors and extensors of the hips.
- Maintaining scapular depression using scapular stabilizers.

Tips
✔ Keep the hips stacked.
✔ Lengthen top arm away from top leg.
✔ Push forearm and elbow into the floor.

(17) SINGLE LEG STRETCH PREP

Start Position

1. Spine imprinted.
2. Sit in front of the BOSU on the mat.
3. Place the lower back against the dome.
4. Upper body is flexed forward.
5. Hands placed on the mat besides the hips.
6. Knees bent slightly apart and parallel.
7. Feet on the mat and in-line with sitting bones.

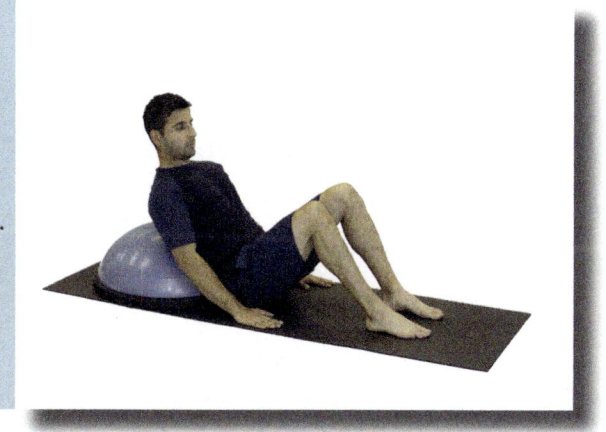

Exercise

Inhale	Push both palms into the floor and lift the R foot off the mat.	
Exhale	Extend R leg out in parallel, hovering above the mat.	
Inhale	Bend the R leg.	

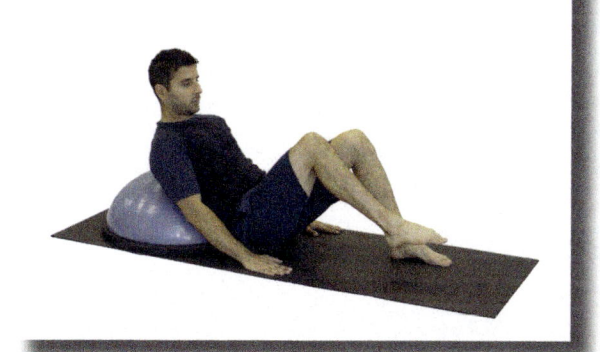

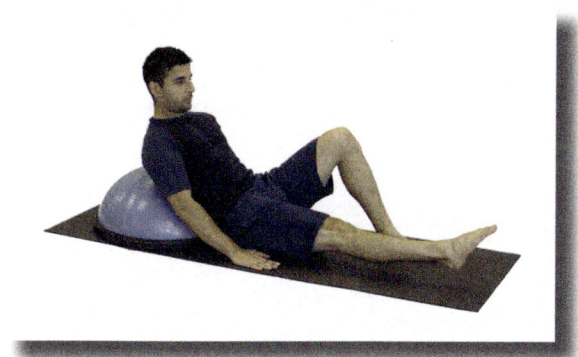

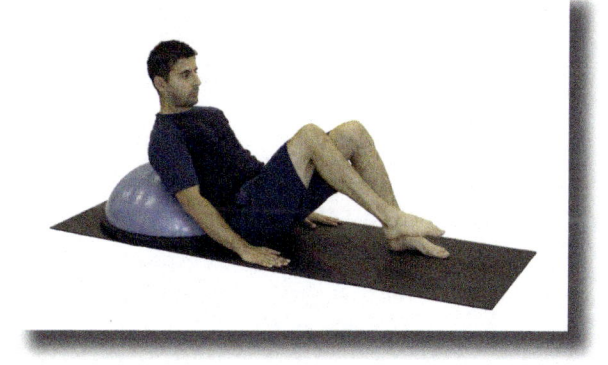

FUNDAMENTALS 55

Exhale   Return to **Start Position.**

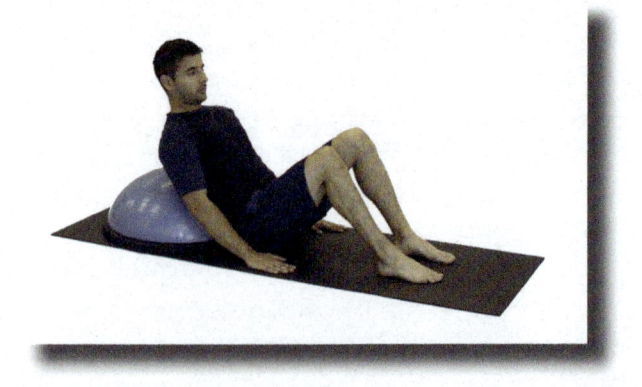

Inhale   Repeating on L leg: Push both palms into the floor and lift the L foot off the mat.

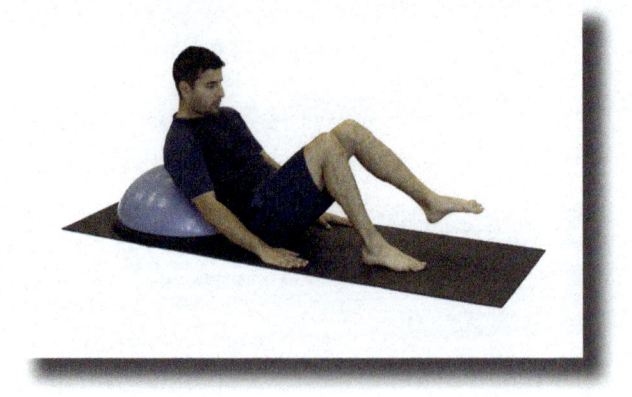

Exhale   Extend L leg out in parallel, hovering above the mat.

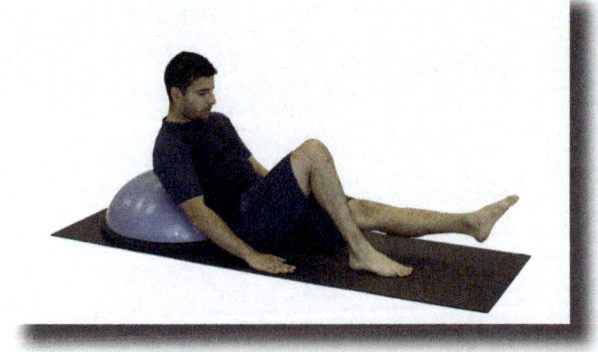

Inhale   Bend the L leg.

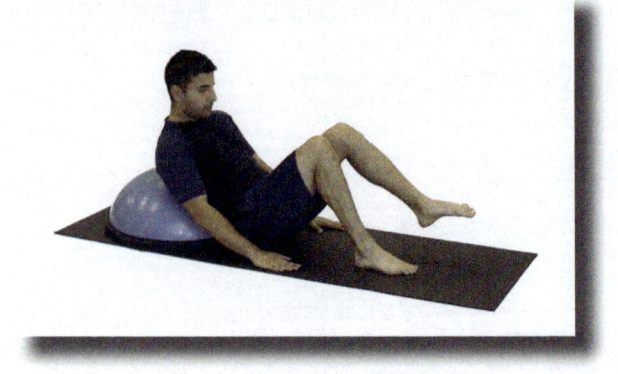

Exhale   Return to **Start Position**.
Reps   X10 Sets

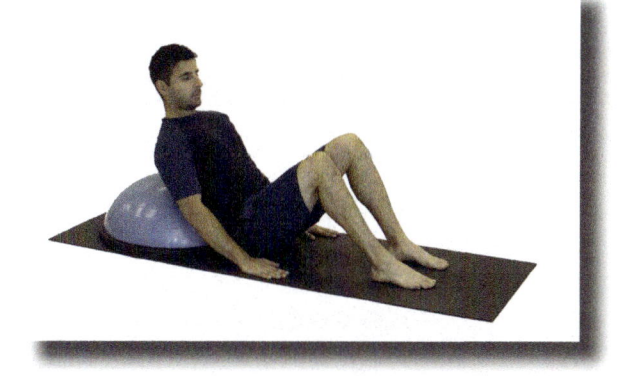

Modified

1. Hands behind the head. Reps X5 Sets. (CHALLENGE)

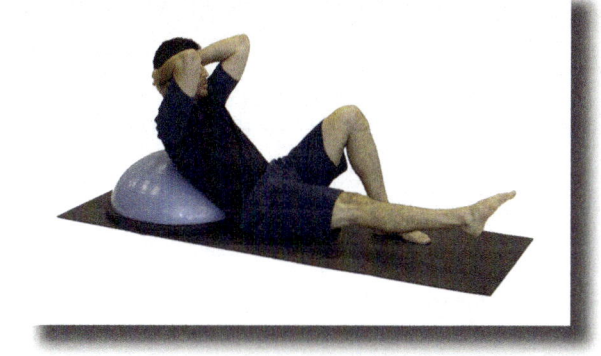

2. Head and shoulders on the mat, hips on top of dome. Extend one leg at a time to the ceiling. Hands hold the mat or the dome. Reps X5 Sets (SIMPLIFY)

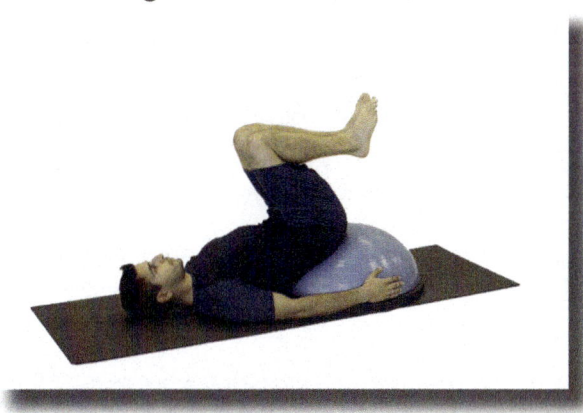

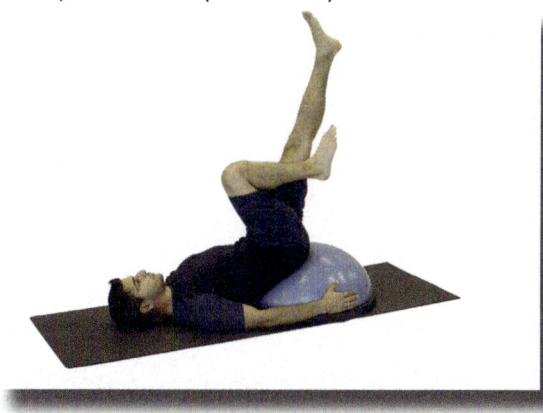

3. Hands behind the head. Extend the R leg, then bring the R knee into the chest X5. Then change sides. (CHALLENGE)

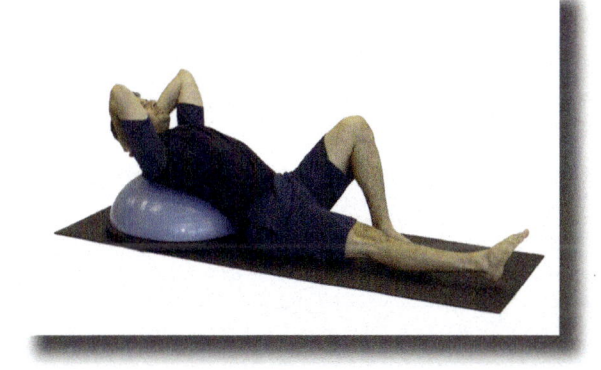

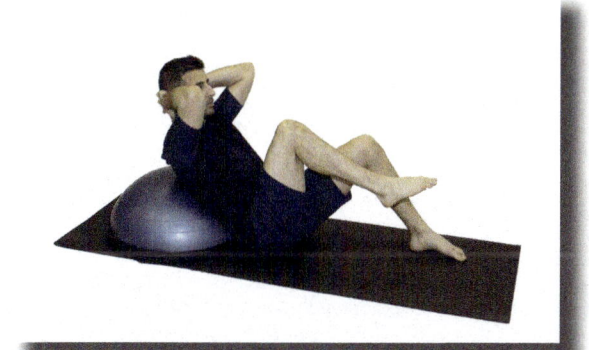

FUNDAMENTALS

4. Deepen the curl forward and alternate the legs keeping the knees bent, placing the foot on the floor in between. Increase speed. Reps X10 (SIMPLIFY)

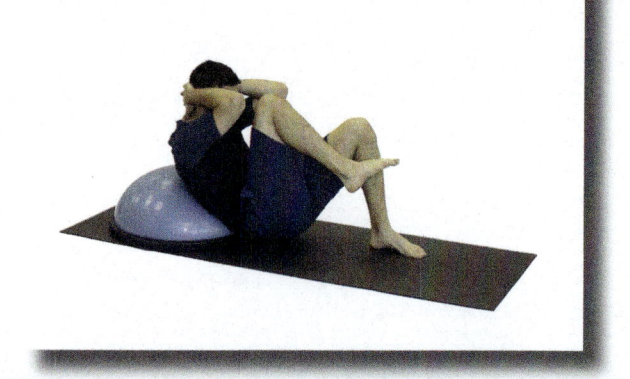

Muscular Intention

- Stabilizing and flexing the spine using abdominals.
- Stabilizing the flexors and extensors of the working hip.
- Maintaining scapular depression using scapular stabilizers.
- Stabilizing pelvis using abdominals, specifically obliques during leg extension and flexion.
- Strengthening the hamstrings, glutes and obliques while pushing the supporting foot into the mat.

Tips

- ✔ Press both hands into the mat while leaning back onto the dome.
- ✔ Slide shoulders down the back.
- ✔ Deepen the abdominal connection with hands behind the head.
- ✔ With hands behind the head, press the head into the hands and hands against the head.

(18) DOUBLE LEG STRETCH PREP

Start Position

1. Spine imprinted.
2. Sit in front of the BOSU on the mat.
3. Place the lower back against the front half of the dome.
4. Upper body is flexed forward.
5. Hands placed on the mat besides the hips.
6. Knees bent slightly apart and parallel.
7. Feet on the mat and in-line with sitting bones.

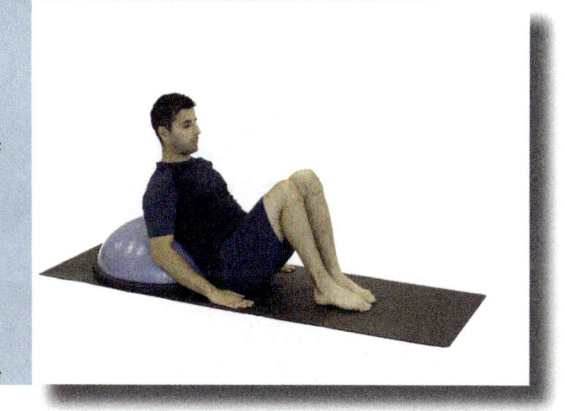

Exercise

Inhale   Extend both legs parallel along the mat.

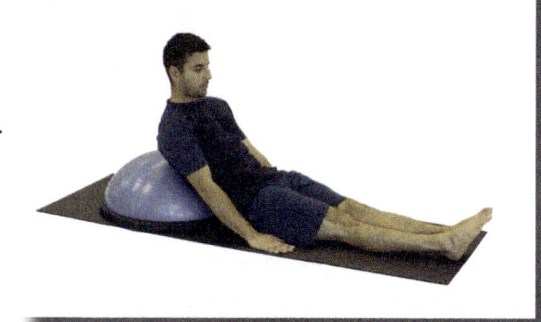

Exhale   Push hands into the mat and bend both knees into the chest, feet off the mat. Place both feet on the floor.

Reps   X10

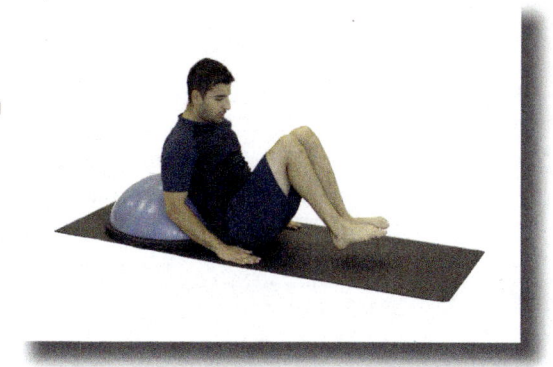

Inhale   Return to **Start Position**.

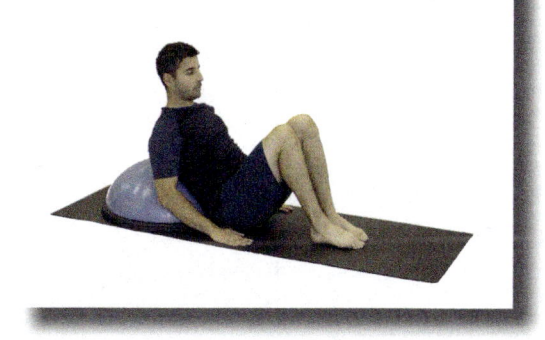

FUNDAMENTALS   59

Modified

1. Hands behind the head – Slide the feet along the mat as you straighten and bend the legs. Reps X10 (CHALLENGE)

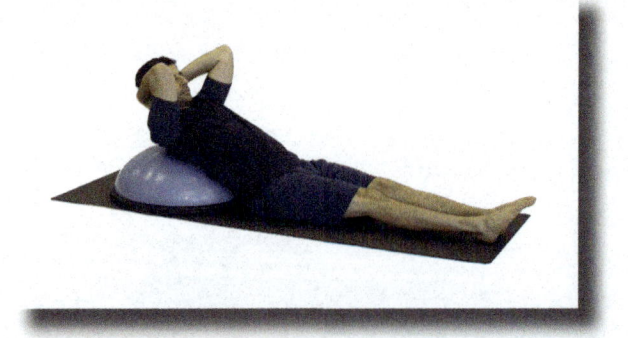

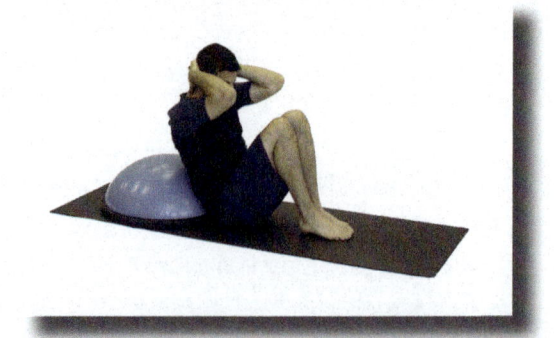

2. Double knee lift. Reps X10 (CHALLENGE)

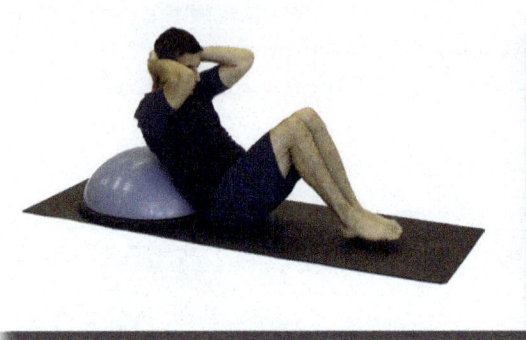

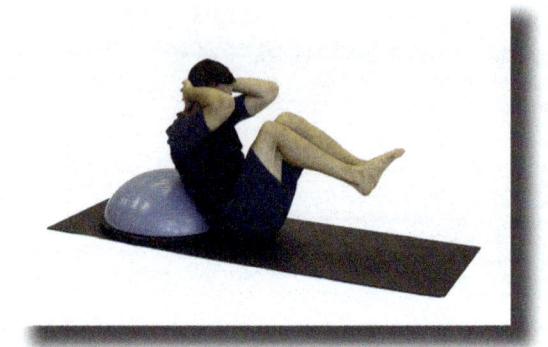

3. Head and shoulders on the mat, hips on top of the dome. Hands hold the mat or dome. Bring the knees toward the chest. Then straighten the legs up to the ceiling. Reps X10 (SIMPLIFY)

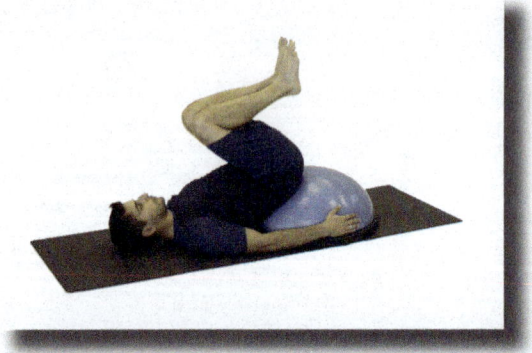

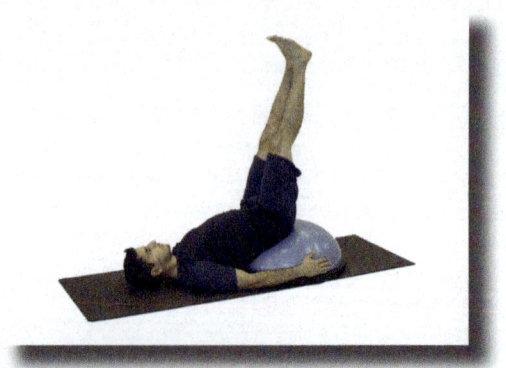

Muscular Intention

- Stabilizing and flexing the spine using abdominals.
- Stabilizing the hamstrings, glutes and obliques while pushing the feet into the mat.
- Maintaining scapular depression using scapular stabilizers.

Tips

- ✔ Stretch the legs fully without hyper extending the knee.
- ✔ Slide shoulders down the back and keep the collar bones wide.
- ✔ Deepen the abdominal connection.
- ✔ Squeeze the inner thighs together.

(19) SCISSORS PREP

Start Position

1. Spine imprinted.
2. Sit in front of the BOSU on the mat.
3. Place the lower back against the dome.
4. Upper body is flexed forward.
5. Hands placed on the mat besides the hips.
6. Both legs are extended and together along the mat.

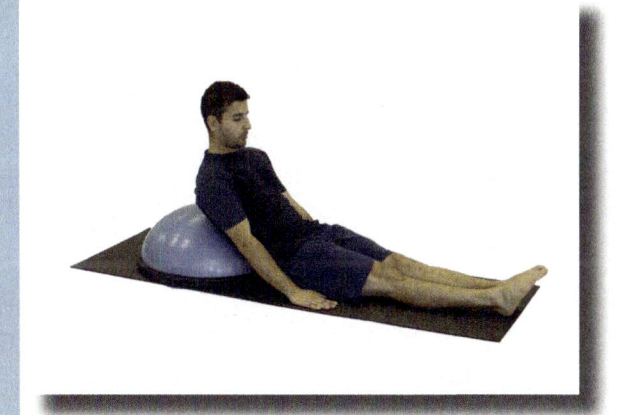

Exercise

Inhale   Engage the abdominals and press both hands into the mat.

Exhale   Extend and lift the L leg. (Two pulses double breath) reaching bottom leg away from body.

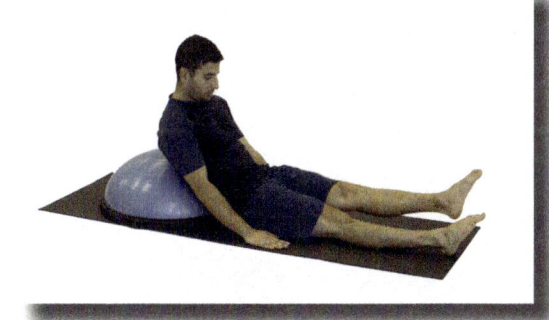

Inhale   Place the L leg down.

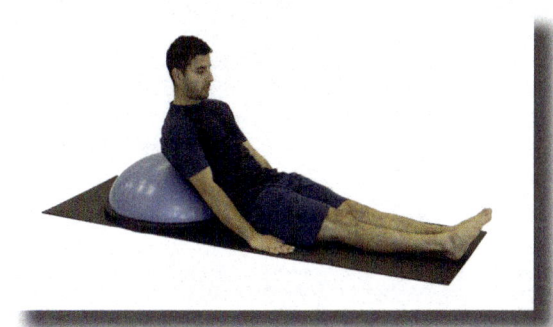

Exhale   Repeat on the R leg. (Two pulses, double breath) reaching bottom leg away from body. Replace the R leg.

Reps   X10 Sets

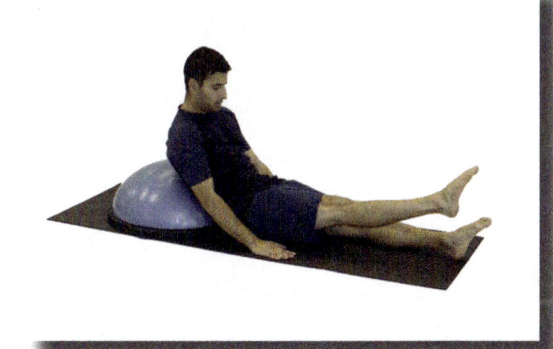

FUNDAMENTALS

Modified

1. Hands behind the head, deepening the abdominal connection. Alternate lifting leg. Reps X10 Sets (SIMPLIFY)

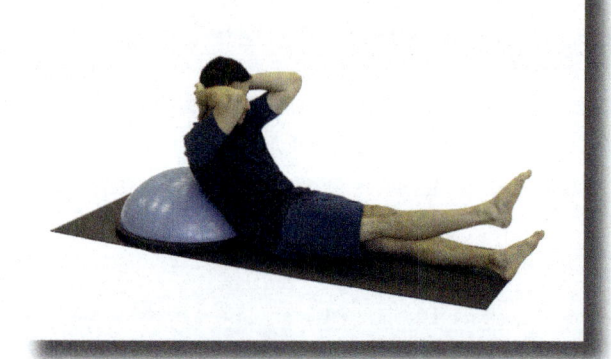

2. Suspend both legs together in midair as you change legs, arms pushing into mat or hands behind the head. Reps X10 Sets (CHALLENGE)

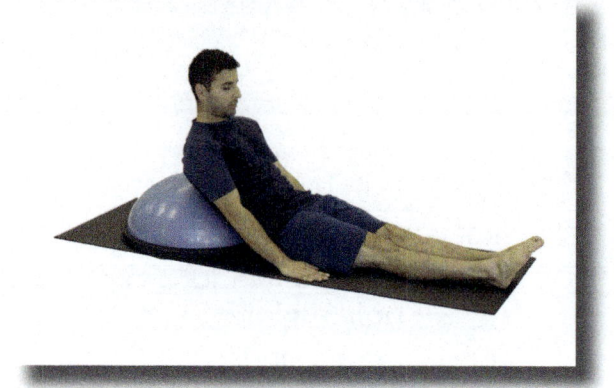

Both legs on the mat.

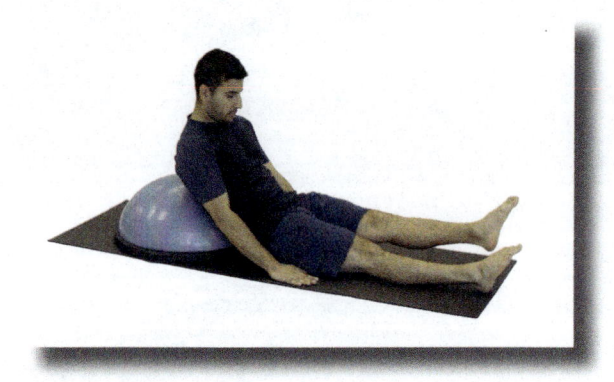

Lift the L leg.

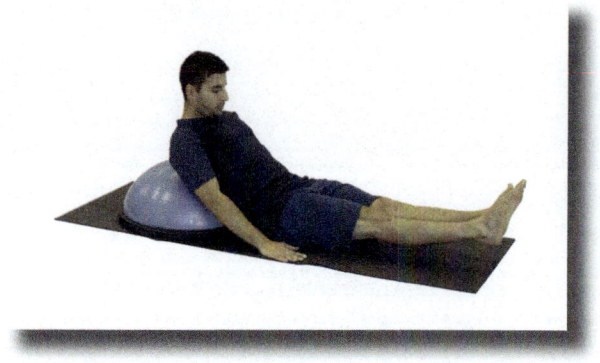

Lift the R leg to meet the L, hovering.

3. Head and shoulders on the mat, hips on top of the dome, hands hold mat or dome. Feet can be pointed or flexed. Reps X10 Sets (SIMPLIFY)

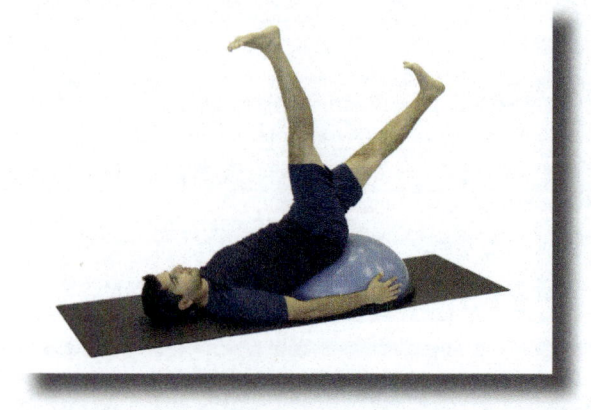

EXERCISES

Muscular Intention

- Stabilizing and flexing the spine using abdominals.
- Stabilizing and strengthening the flexors and extensors of the hips.
- Maintaining scapular depression using scapular stabilizers.
- Stabilizing pelvis using abdominals, specifically obliques during leg extension and flexion.
- Stabilizing the hamstrings, glutes and obliques while pushing the bottom leg into the mat.

Tips

- ✔ Maintain lower back pressing into dome using lower abdominals.
- ✔ Fully extending the back of the knees along the mat.
- ✔ Slide shoulders down the back and keep the collar bones wide.
- ✔ Only lower the leg as low as the abdominals can control.

FUNDAMENTALS

(20) SHOULDER BRIDGE PREP

Start Position

1. Spine imprinted.
2. Head and shoulders on the dome.
3. Hips on the mat.
4. Knees bent slightly apart and parallel.
5. Feet on the mat and in-line with sitting bones.
6. Hands on the hips, or alone the mat.

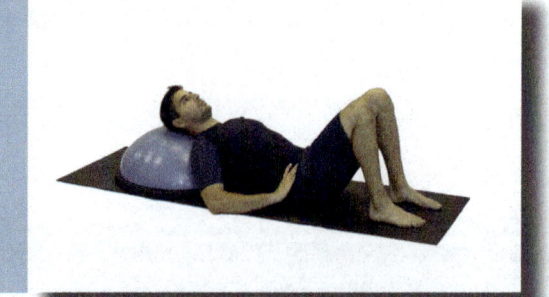

Exercise

Inhale   Lengthen the spine.

Exhale   Push into both feet as you curl the pelvis and roll through the spine into shoulder bridge.

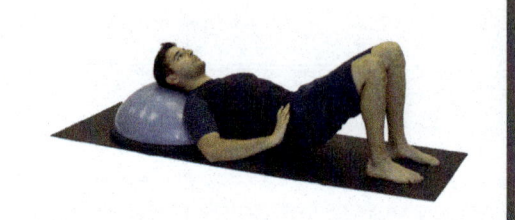

Inhale   Hold the bridge position.

Exhale   Lift L leg to tabletop. Push into the floor with the R foot.

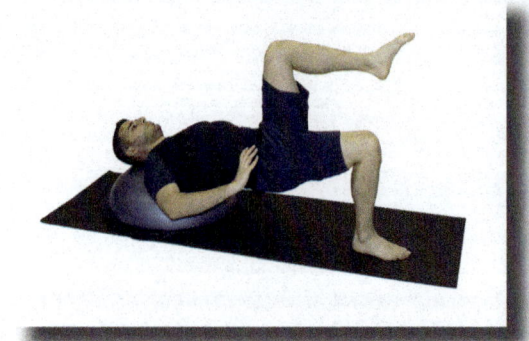

Inhale   Lower the L foot return to mat. Hands on hips.

»   Repeat with R leg.

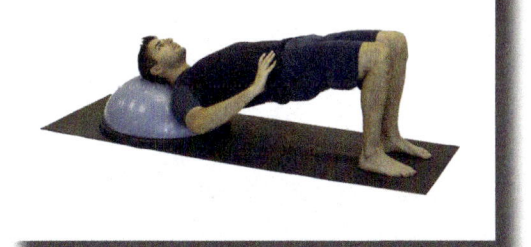

To Finish...

Exhale   Hold the bridge, lifting hips even higher.

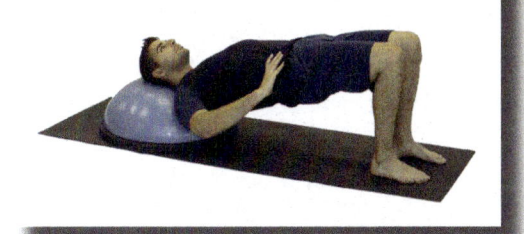

Inhale   Roll down one vertebra at a time lengthening spine to **Start Position**.
Reps   X5-10 Sets

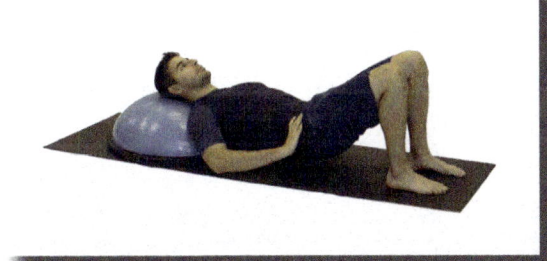

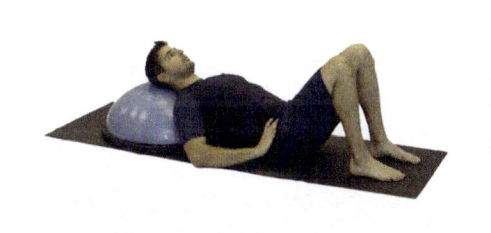

Modified

1. Head and shoulders on the dome. Hips in bridge position. Lift and lower both heels. Reps X10 (SIMPLIFY)

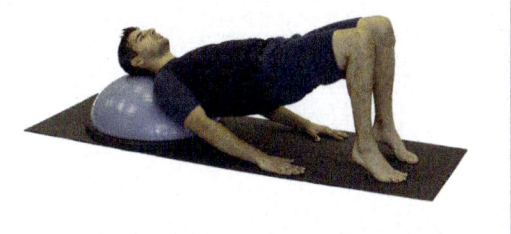

2. Lift and lower the toes. Reps X10 (SIMPLIFY)

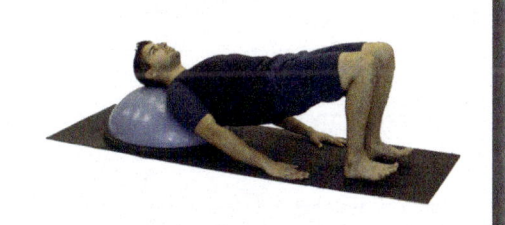

FUNDAMENTALS

3. Lower and lift hips with spinal articulation. Reps X10 (SIMPLIFY)

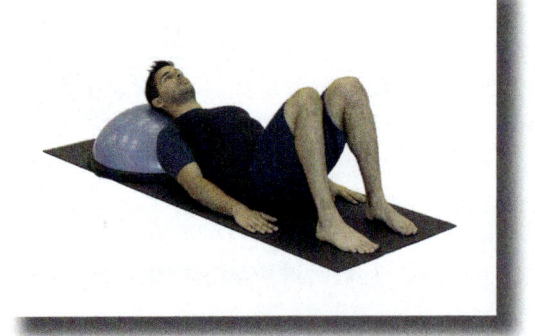

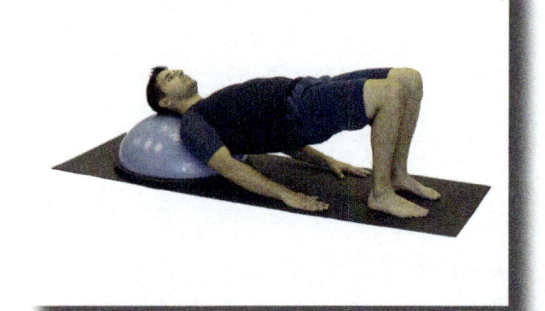

4. Place the head and shoulders on the mat and hips on top of the dome. Push down into L foot and squeeze the L glute. Lift R foot to tabletop. Unfold the R leg straight up to the ceiling. Reps X5 L/R (SIMPLIFY)

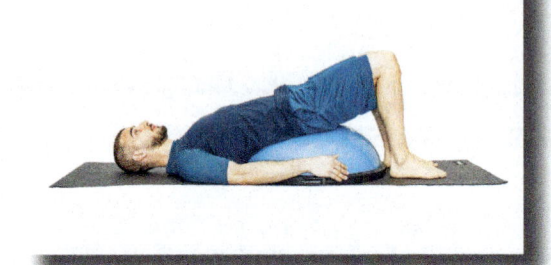

Feet on the floor.

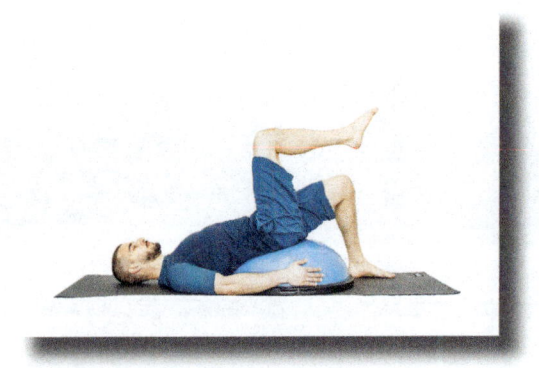

Lift the right knee to tabletop.

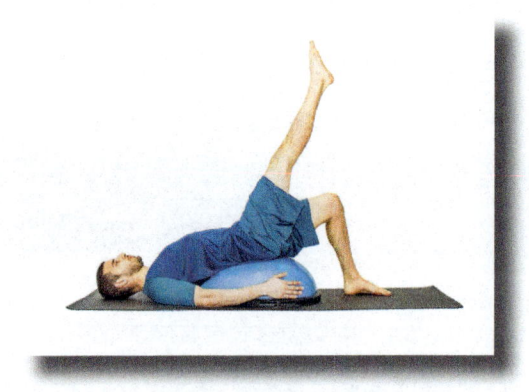

Unfold the R leg straight up to the ceiling.

5. Hold the shoulder bridge, and alternate single heel and toe lift. X5 L/R (CHALLENGE)

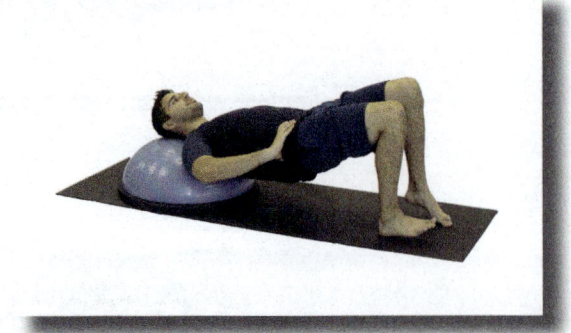

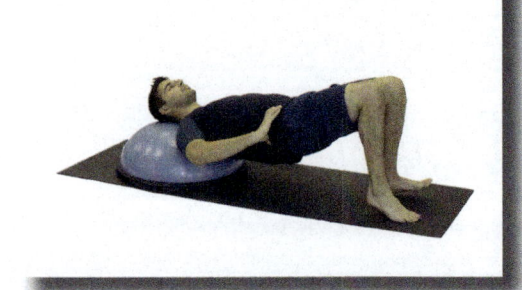

66 EXERCISES

Muscular Intention

- Releasing and mobilizing the full spine during the curl into the bridge.
- Connecting to the deep abdominals during forward flexion and the paraspinals in extension.
- Stabilizing the hamstrings, glutes and obliques while pushing the feet into the mat.

Tips

- ✔ Relax the quadriceps.
- ✔ Maintain fluidity during the pelvic tilt.
- ✔ Slide the shoulders down the back to lengthen the neck.
- ✔ Keep the feet and knees in line with the sitting bones.
- ✔ Push down into both feet to lift the hips and simultaneously send the tailbone forward.

(21) ROLL OVER PREP

Start Position

1. Spine imprinted.
2. Head and shoulders on the mat.
3. Hips on top of the dome.
4. Knees bent 90° and hips bent 90°.
5. Legs together.
6. Arms at the sides, holding the dome.

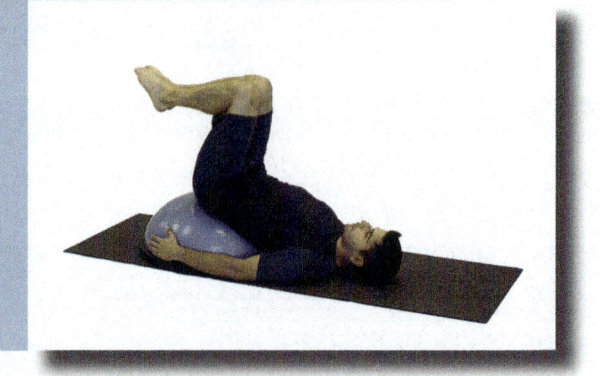

Exercise

Inhale	Imprint the lower spine and bring bent knees to the chest.
Exhale	Lift the hips off the BOSU.
Inhale	Hold this position with hips up.
Exhale	Sequentially roll back onto the BOSU with bent knees. Return to **Start Position.**
Reps	X5-10

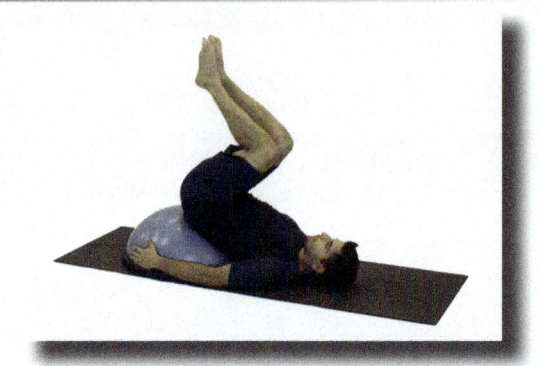

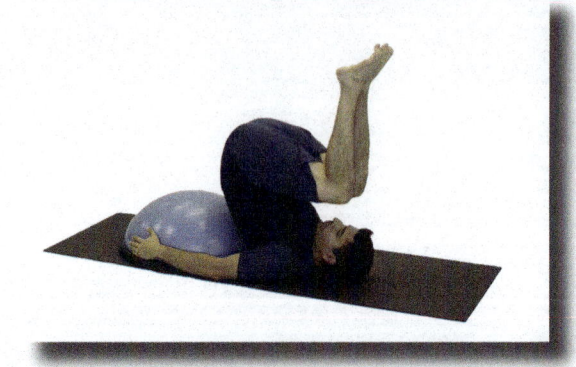

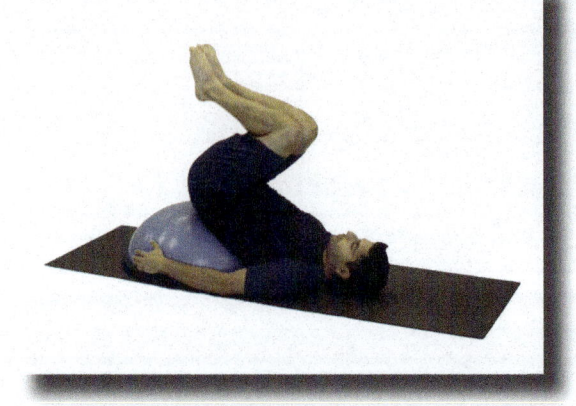

68 EXERCISES

Modified

1. Practice straight legs to the ceiling and bring the knees to the chest, rolling hips off and onto the dome. Hands hold the dome. Reps X5-10 (ASSIST)

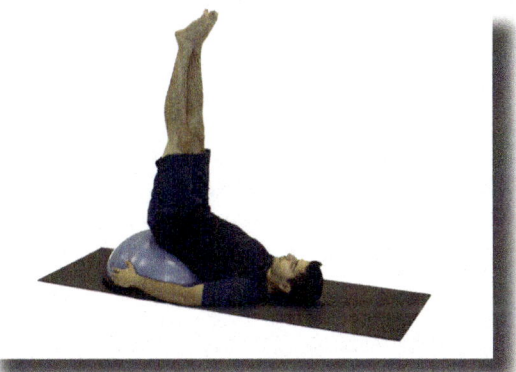

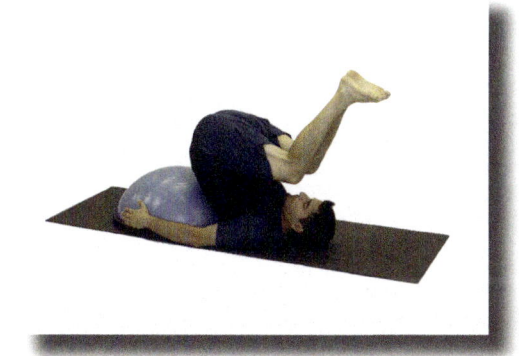

2. Head, shoulders and torso on the mat. Hands hold the sides of the dome overhead. Knees bent, to table top. Bring bent knees to chest and lift hips off the mat. Keeping knees bent, roll the hips back down. Reps X5-10 (CHALLENGE)

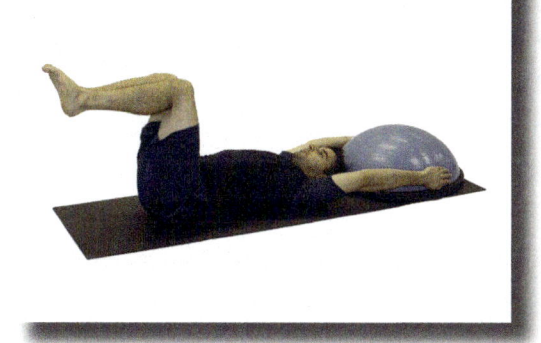

Muscular Intention

- Contracting the abdominals to initiate the roll over.
- Stabilizing the deep core muscles specifically the obliques and transverse abdominus.
- Maintaining scapular depression using scapular stabilizers.
- Connecting the arms by hugging the BOSU through the back using the full core muscles.

Tips

- ✔ Slide the shoulders down the back and keep the collar bones wide.
- ✔ Roll onto the shoulders, not the neck
- ✔ Control the roll up and the roll down using the lower abdominals.

FUNDAMENTALS

(22) DOUBLE LEG EXTENSION PREP

Start Position

1. Pelvis imprinted.
2. Prone, belly on top of the dome.
3. Elbows flexed, forearms on the mat, hands clasped.
4. Head and neck extended.
5. Legs slightly apart, extended and parallel.
6. Feet flexed with toes tucked under.

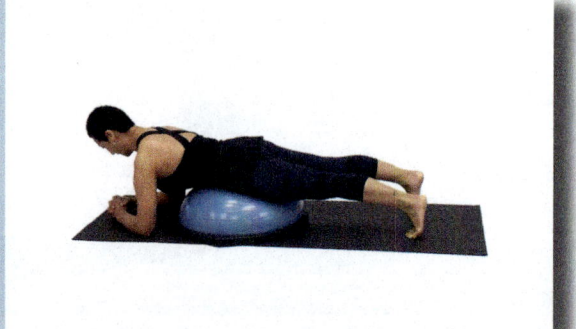

Exercise

Inhale   To lengthen the spine.

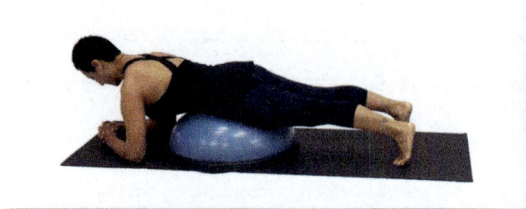

Exhale   Engage the lower abdominals, extend and lift both legs to hip height, feet pointed.

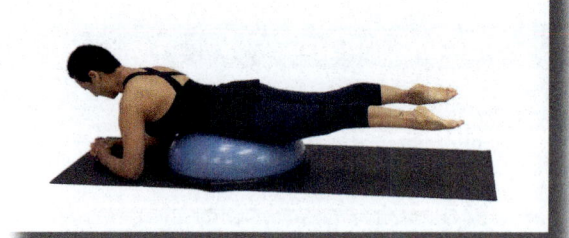

Inhale   Lower the legs and return feet to flexed on mat.

Reps   X5-10

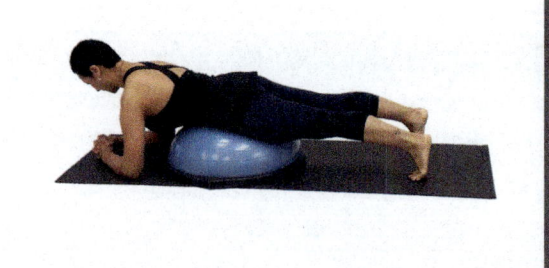

Modified

1. Extend and lift one leg at a time. Reps 5-10 L/R (ASSIST)
2. Circle extended legs CCW and CW. Do not buckle at the knees, circle from hamstrings and glutes. Reps X10 CW/CCW L/R (CHALLENGE)

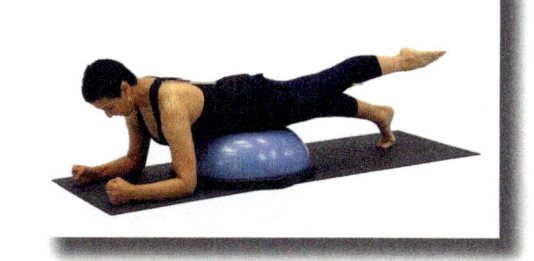

3. Pulse extended legs upwards. Legs apart or together. Reps X10 (CHALLENGE)

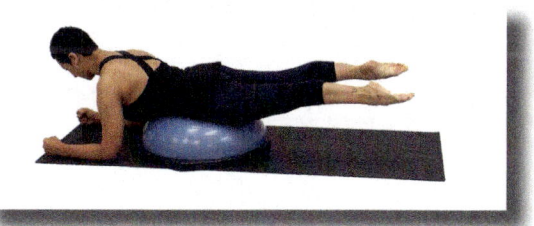

4. Knees and feet on the mat. Bend and stretch both knees only. Feet can be flexed or pointed. Reps X10 (SIMPLIFY)

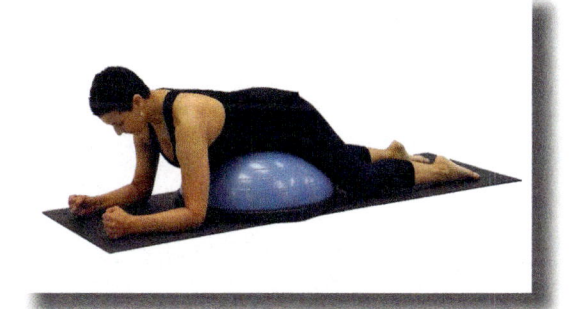

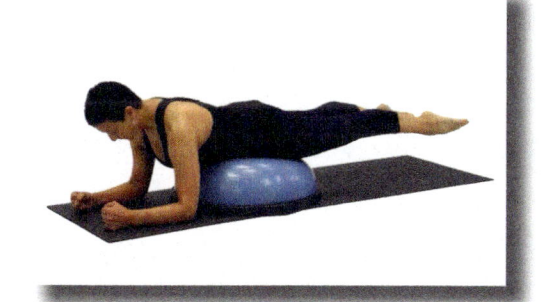

5. Legs hovering, flex and point both feet. Reps X10 (CHALLENGE)

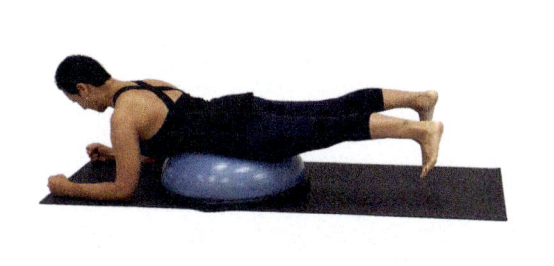

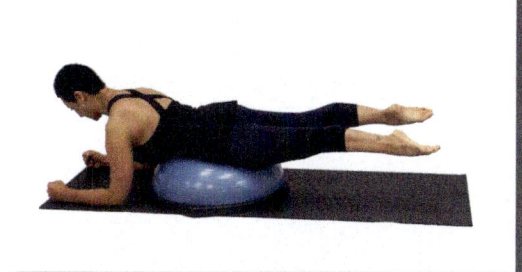

6. Hands clasped or in a fist apart, beat the legs together in extension. Reps X10 (CHALLENGE)

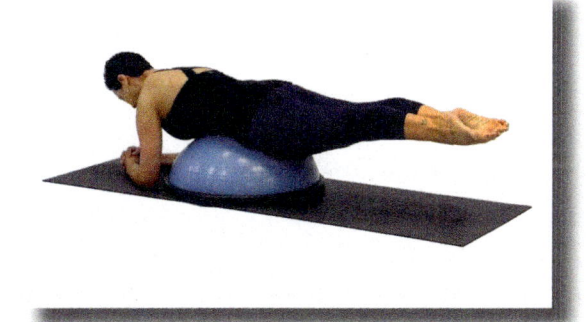

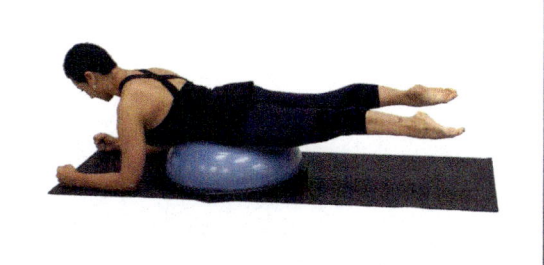

FUNDAMENTALS

Muscular Intention

- Emphasizing mid-thoracic spine during extension.
- Lengthening of the latissimus dorsi and paraspinals.
- Maintaining scapular depression using scapular stabilizers.
- Supporting spine using abdominals.
- Straightening the legs using glutes and hamstrings.

Tips

- ✔ Keep collar bones wide and keep the chin away from the chest.
- ✔ Engage the abdominals throughout.
- ✔ Lengthen the head away from the feet.
- ✔ Lift the legs using the glutes and hamstrings.

(23) SINGLE LEG KICK

Start Position

1. Pelvis imprinted.
2. Prone, belly on the dome.
3. Supporting upper body on elbows, hands in fists.
4. Legs extended and slightly apart.
5. Feet flexed with toes tucked under.
6. Head in line with the spine.

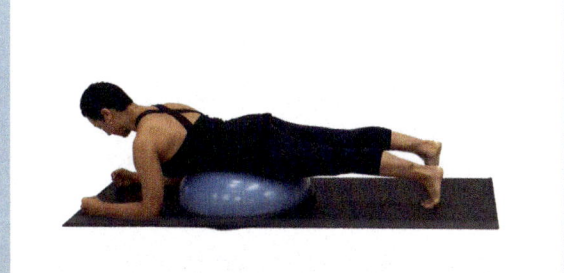

Exercise

Inhale — Lengthen and lift the L leg.

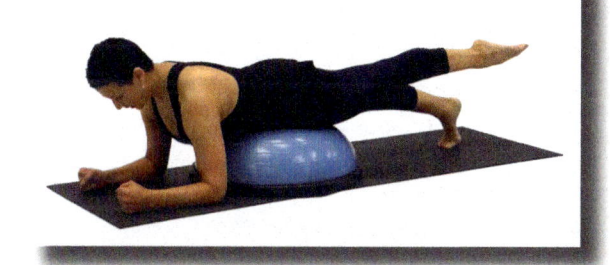

Exhale — Bend the L knee with foot pointed for one beat then beat 3 times toward the pelvis with foot flexed. Point the foot, keeping the leg bent, increasing the glute connection by lifting the knee higher.

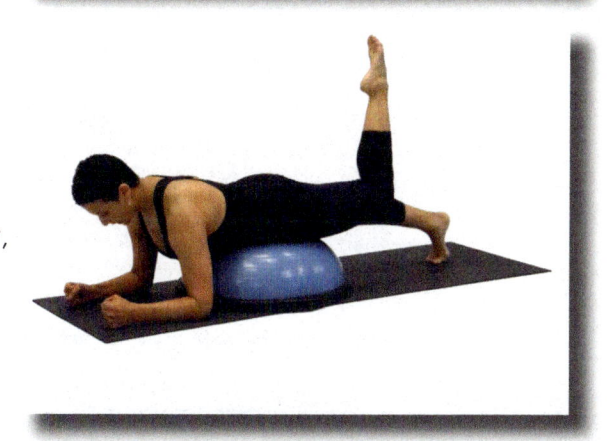

Bend the L knee with foot pointed for one beat.

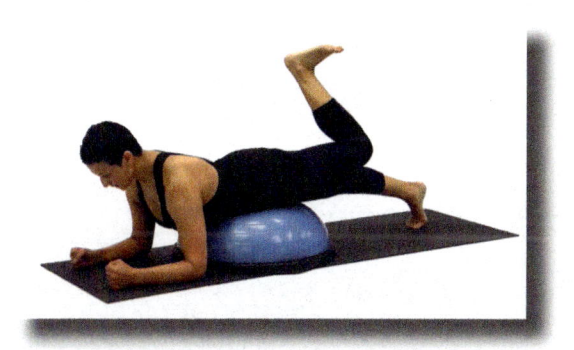

3 beats with the foot flexed.

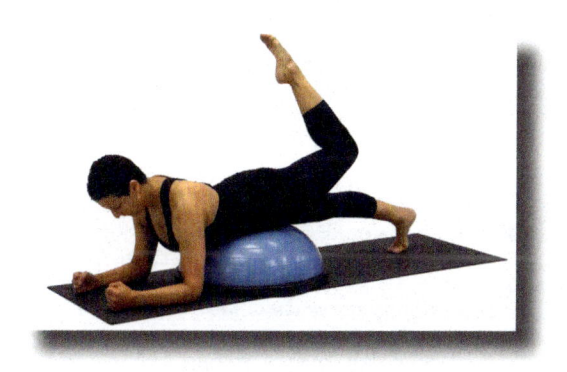

Lifting the knee higher.

FUNDAMENTALS 73

Inhale   Extend L knee with foot pointed and extend the L hip slightly to reach the leg away.

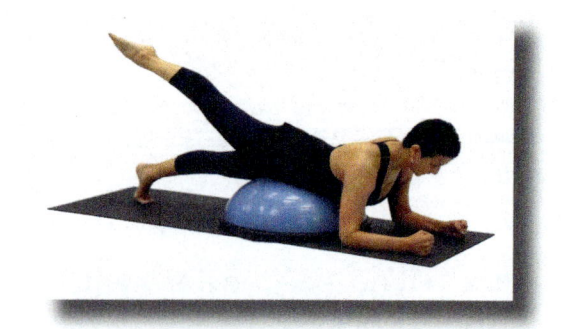

Exhale   Return foot to **Start Position**.
Reps   X5

» Repeat on R leg.

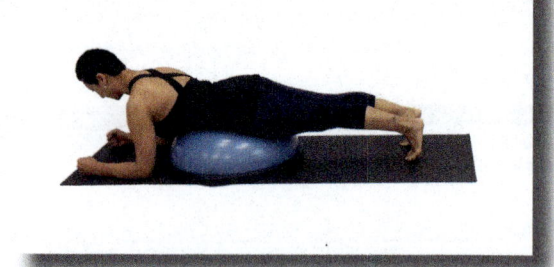

Modified
1. Forearm position: Hands in fists on mat. Bend the knee to pulse L heel to ceiling. Reps X10 L/R (SIMPLIFY)

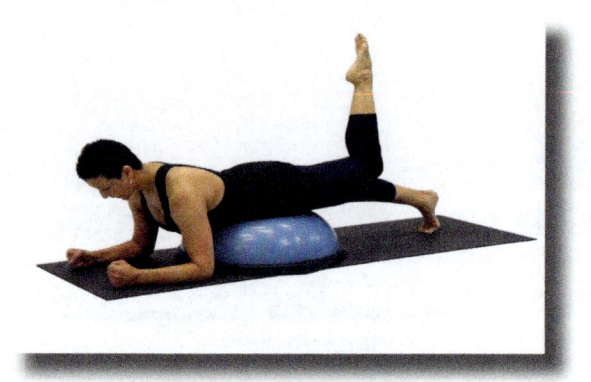

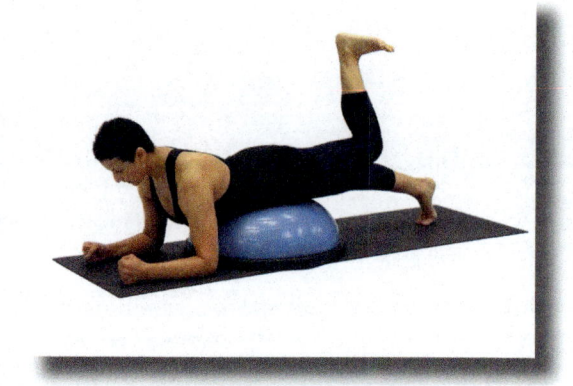

Muscular Intention
- Emphasizing mid-thoracic spine during extension.
- Lengthening and strengthening of the latissimus dorsi and paraspinals.
- Maintaining scapular depression using scapular stabilizers.
- Supporting the spine using abdominals.
- Straightening the legs using glutes and hamstrings.
- Lengthening the quadriceps especially while bending the knee.

Tips
- ✔ Deepen the lower abdominals throughout.
- ✔ Use the glutes and hamstrings to lift and bend the knee.
- ✔ Lengthen the head away from the feet in extension.
- ✔ Press the forearms into the mat while pulling shoulders down the back.

(24) SAW

Start Position

1. Spine neutral.
2. Sit on top of dome.
3. Legs extended, wider than hip width apart.
4. Feet flexed.
5. Arms extended out to the sides at shoulder height.
6. Palms facing down.

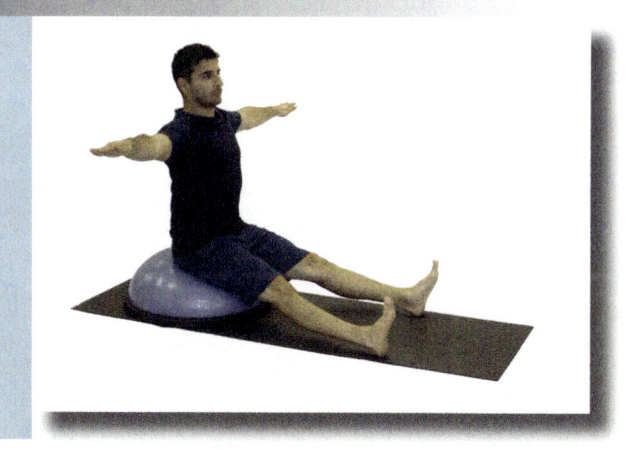

Exercise

Inhale   Rotate the spine R to face the sidewall, hips stay square to the front, while rotating the palms forward.

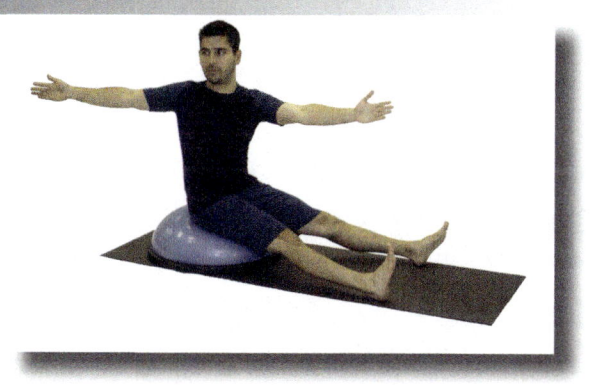

Exhale   Engage the low abdominals and reach L hand fingers toward the baby toe of R foot - curve upper spine. R arm medially rotates and reaches as far back as possible.

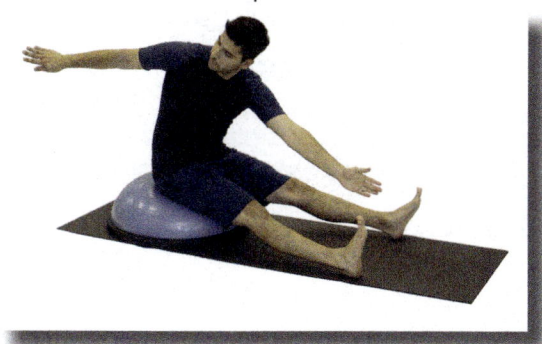

Rotate and deepen the curve.

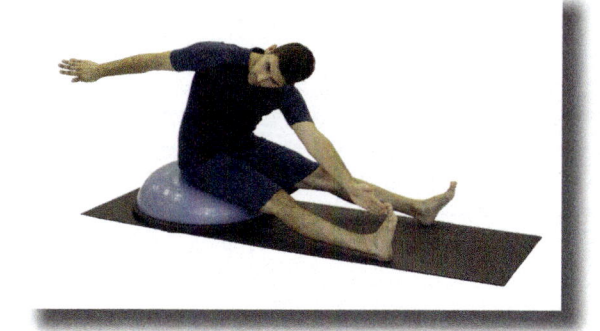

Increase the curve and reach for the baby toe.

FUNDAMENTALS 75

Inhale   Roll up through each vertebra increasing the spine rotation while laterally rotating R arm and palms to face forward.

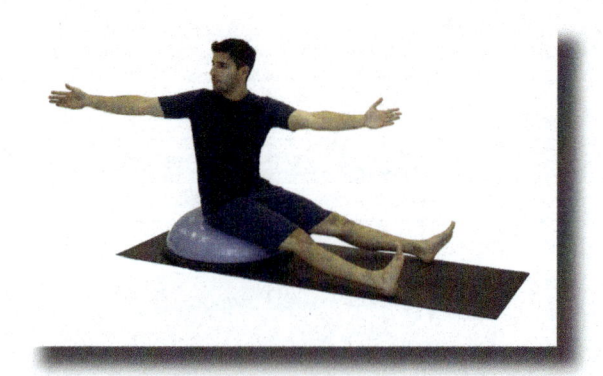

Exhale   Return the spine to **Start Position**, palms down.
Reps   X5 L/R

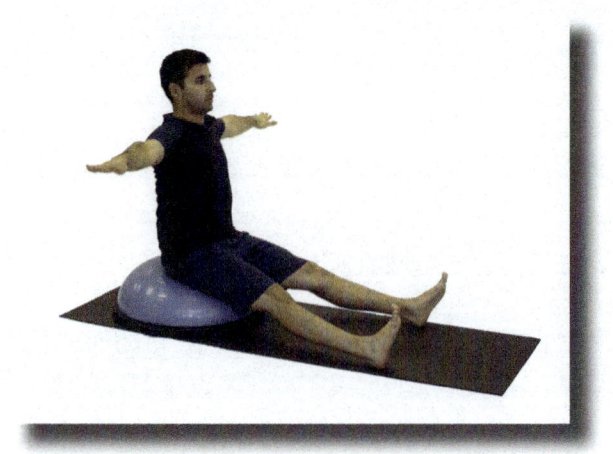

Modified

1. Bend both knees, feet on mat.
   Reps X5 L/R (ASSIST)

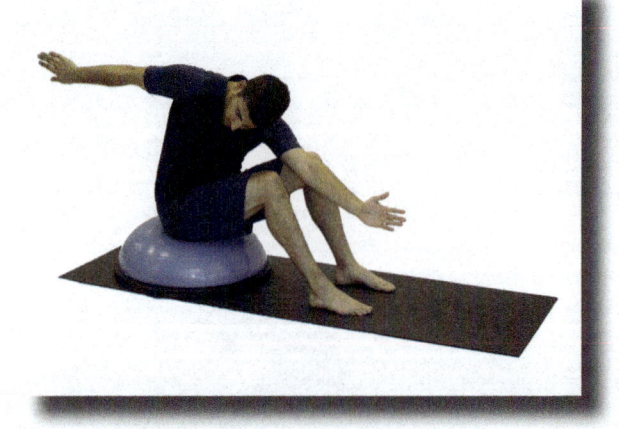

2. R straight leg, L bent knee, reaching toward the straight R leg.
   Reps X5 L/R (ASSIST)

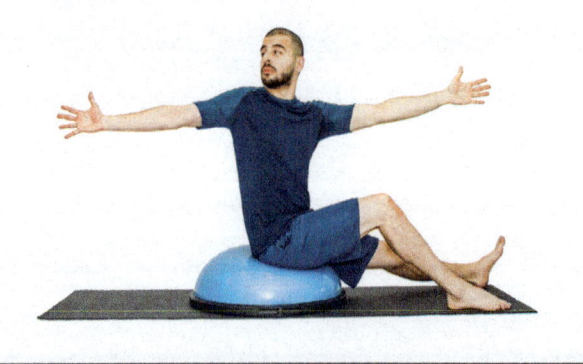

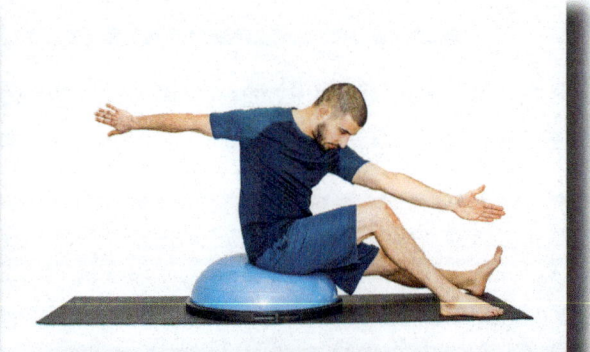

76   **EXERCISES**

3. Flat side up. Do full exercise.
   X5 L/R (CHALLENGE)

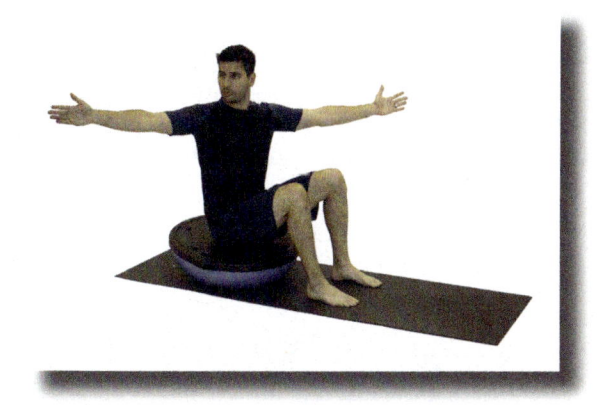

Muscular Intention

- Stabilizing the arms using latissimus dorsi, rhomboids, and teres major.
- Increasing the length in the cervical spine using the deep paraspinals.
- Rotating the spine using obliques and paraspinals.
- Maintaining scapular depression using scapular stabilizers.
- Increasing the action of flexion/rotation using the obliques.
- Rotating the spine using the obliques and paraspinals.

Tips

✔ Maintain neutral pelvis throughout the twist.
✔ Deepen the abdominal connection
✔ Slide the shoulders down the back and keep the collar bones wide.
✔ Increase the length of the spine as you rotate.
✔ Stretch the arms wide across the back.
✔ Stay on both sitting bones during rotation.

FUNDAMENTALS

(25) NECK PULL PREP

Start Position

1. Spine neutral.
2. Sit on the top front half of the dome.
3. Hands behind the head.
4. Knees bent, aligned with the sitting bones.
5. Feet parallel.

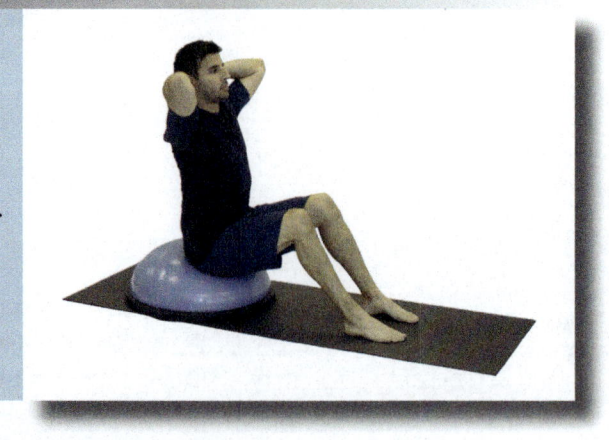

Exercise

Inhale   Lengthen the spine and hinge at the hips.

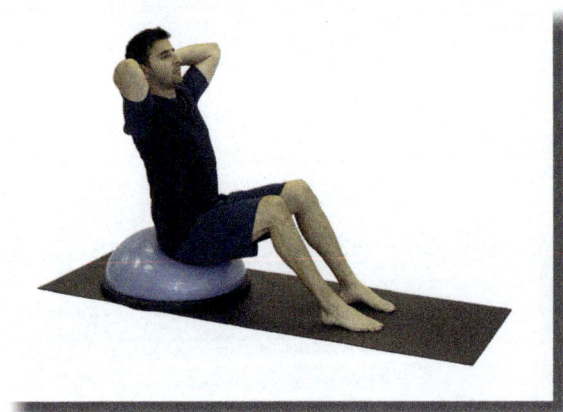

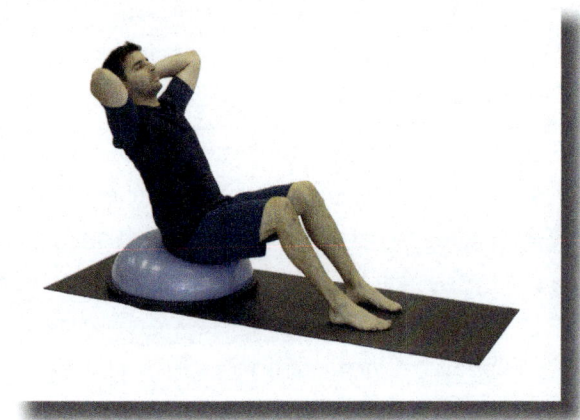

Exhale   Roll back off the sitting bones into posterior pelvic tilt.

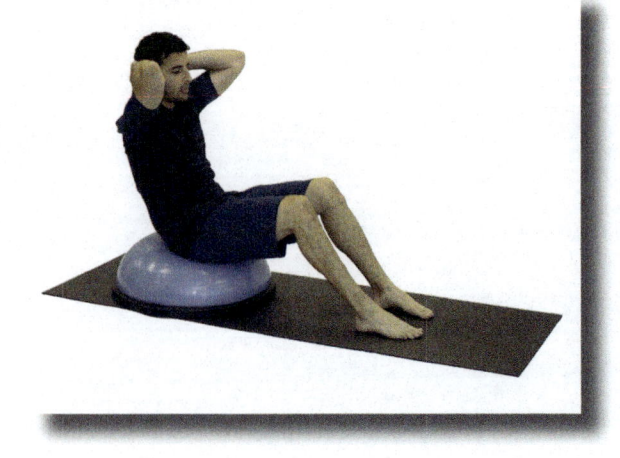

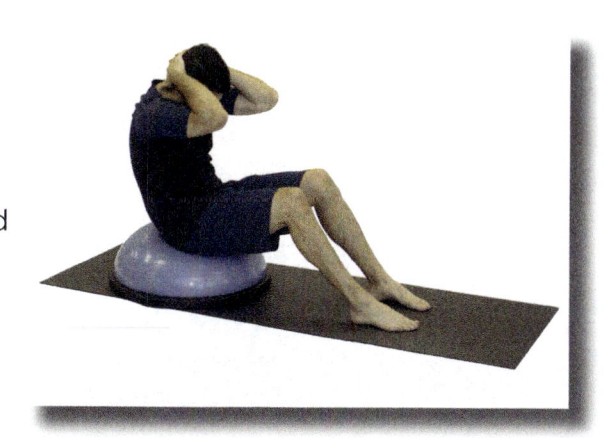

Inhale   Continue to curl forward to a flexed spine.

Exhale   Finish the roll forward and deepen the abdominal curl.

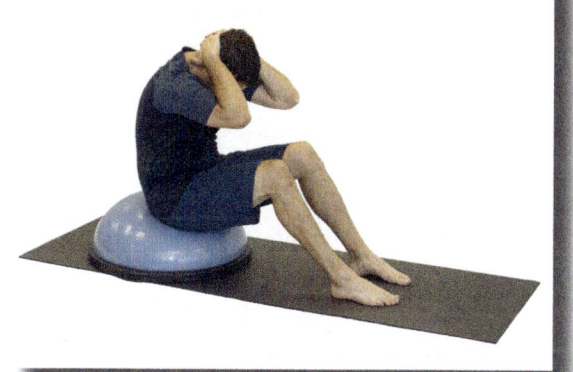

Inhale   Extend the spine back to **Start Position**.
Reps   X5

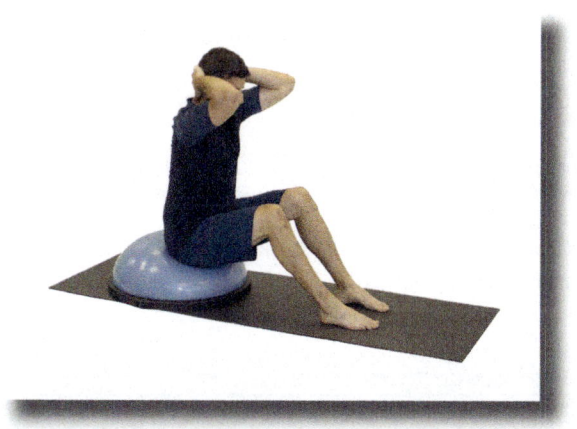

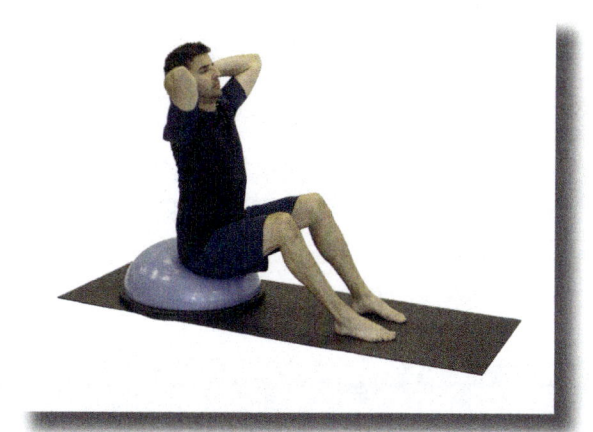

Modified

1. Sit on the mat in front of the BOSU (hands can be in front of head). Reps X5 (ASSIST)

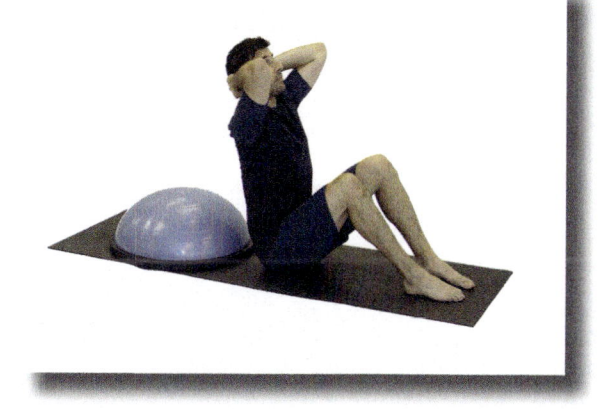

FUNDAMENTALS   79

2. Sit in front of the BOSU and reach the arms forward. Practice the hinge only. Keep the spine straight as you touch the lower back to the dome. Reps X5 (ASSIST)

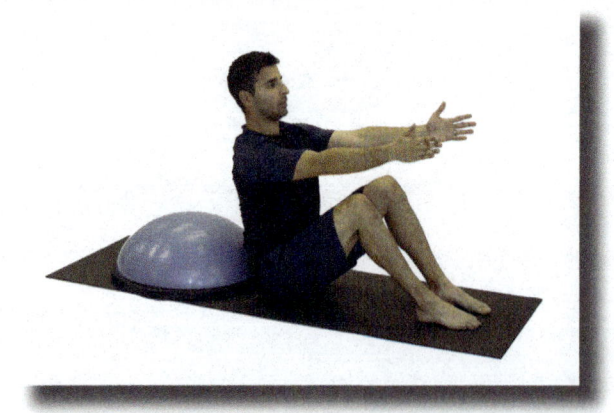

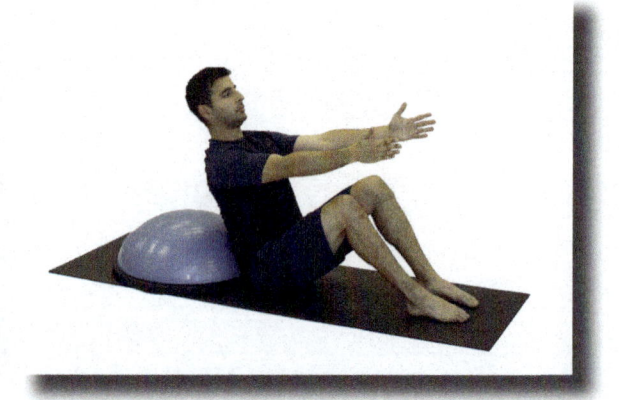

3. Sitting on the top of the dome, do hinge only. Reps X5 (CHALLENGE)

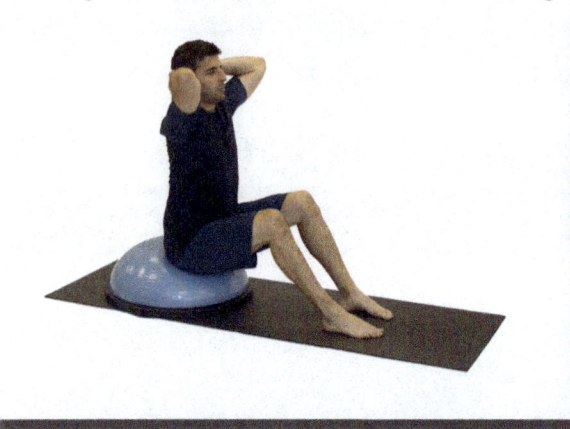

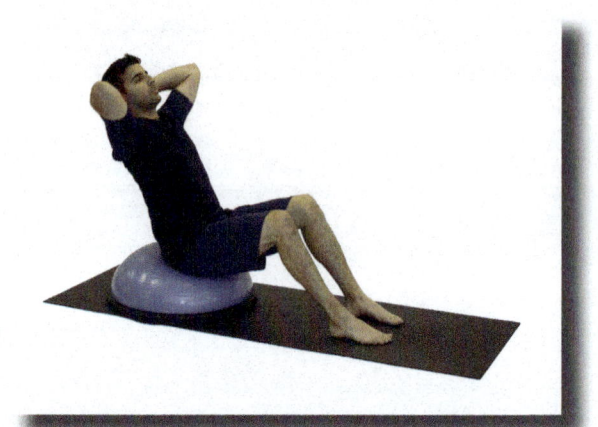

Muscular Intention
- Maintaining scapular depression using scapular stabilizers.
- Engaging the hamstrings and lower glutes.
- Working the deep transverse abdominals and internal obliques.
- Using all abdominals and paraspinals during the hinge.

Tips
- ✔ Increase the length of the spine as you hinge back.
- ✔ Press the head into hands and hands into the head.
- ✔ Slide the shoulders down the back and keep the collar bones wide.
- ✔ Maintain neutral pelvis throughout.

(26) OBLIQUES ROLL BACK

Start Position

1. Spine neutral.
2. Sitting in front of the BOSU.
3. Knees bent, slightly apart.
4. Feet on the mat, in line with sitting bones.
5. Reaching R hand forward at shoulder height palm facing in.
6. Place the L hand behind the head.

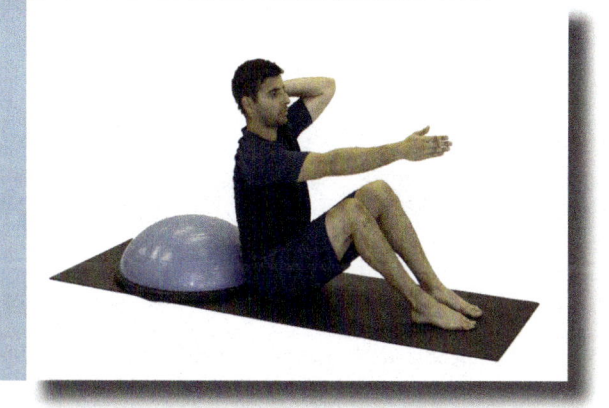

Exercise

Inhale   To deepen the lower spine curl and roll off sitting bones.

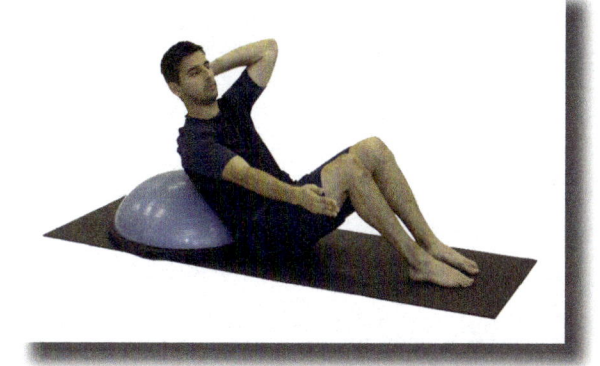

Exhale   Increase the curl as you rotate the spine, reaching R hand down then back toward the back R corner of the room.

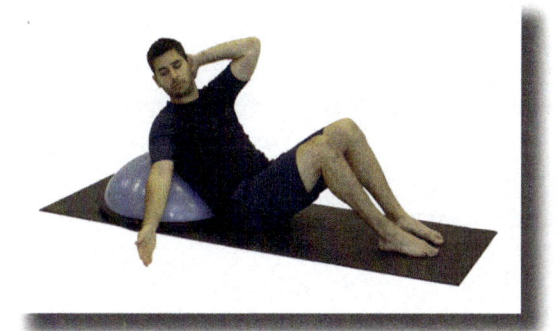

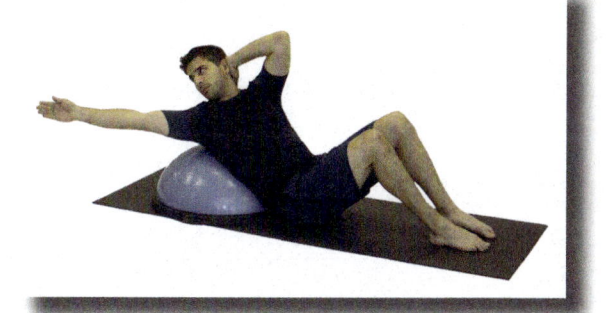

Inhale   Reach the R arm further and lift elbow to ceiling. Gaze in line with straight arm.

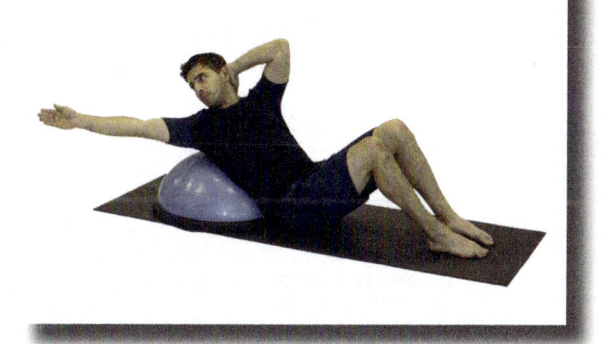

FUNDAMENTALS | 81

Modified

1. Reach both arms to one side. Feet and knees slightly apart. Reps X10 L/R (SIMPLIFY)
2. Knees and feet together. Reps X10 L/R (CHALLENGE)

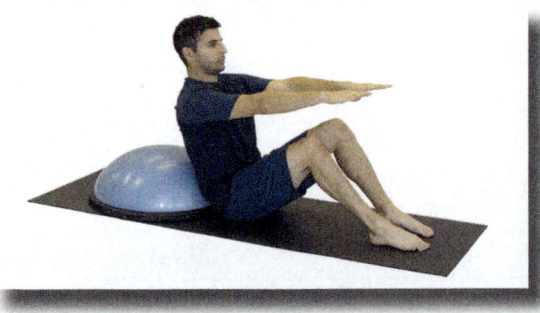

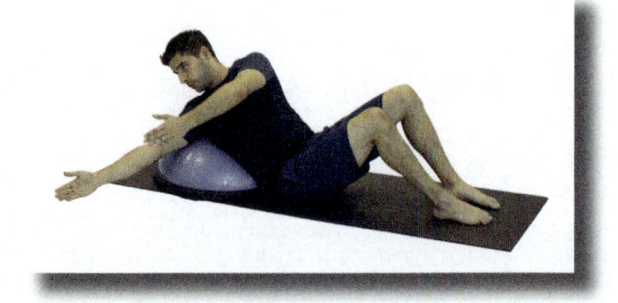

3. Swing the R arm down to floor and then reach the R arm to the back. Follow the hand with your eyes. Return to **Start Position** and alternate sides.
Reps X10 L/R (SIMPLIFY)

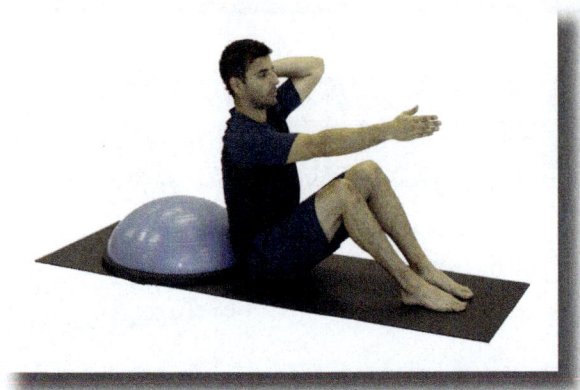

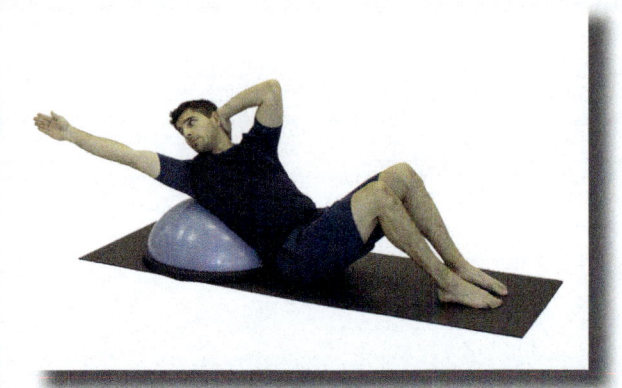

Exhale   Increase the twist in the upper trunk to deepen the abdominal connection (pulsing for 10 counts).

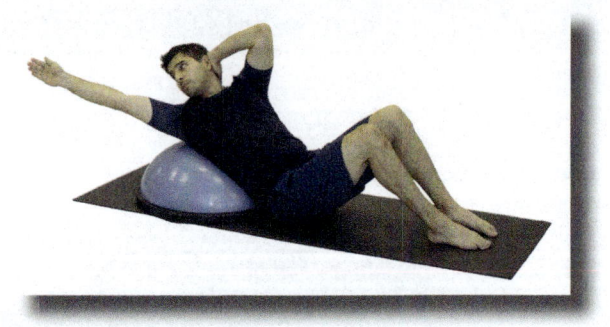

Inhale   Swing the arm down and return to **Start Position**.
Reps   X10 L/R

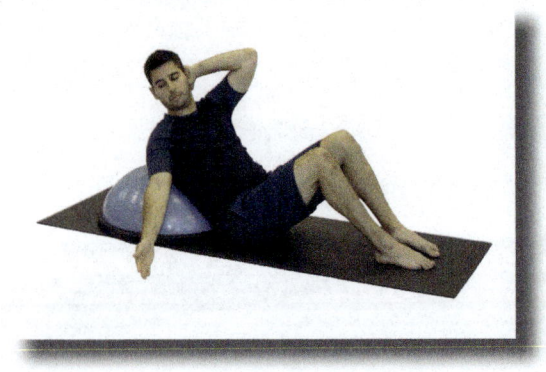

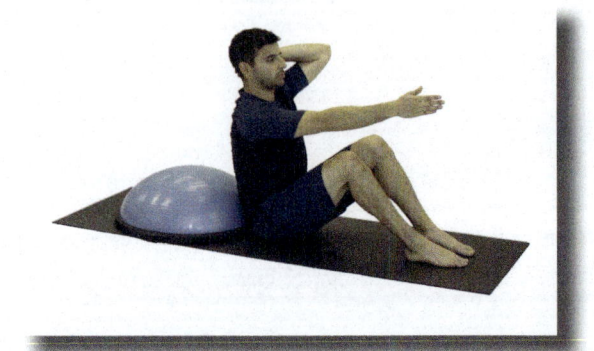

82   **EXERCISES**

Muscular Intention

- Using the obliques to draw the rib cage across and toward the opposite hip.
- Stabilizing the pelvis and flexing the spine using abdominals.
- Stabilizing the legs using hamstrings and glutes.

Tips

✔ Slide the shoulders down the back and keep the collar bones wide.
✔ Reaching the elbow toward the ceiling while reaching the other arm out and long.
✔ Keep both sides of the rib cage straight and long. (Stay centre of your spine.)
✔ Keep both sitting bones on the mat.

(27) TEASER PREP

Start Position

1. Spine imprinted.
2. Sitting at the front of the BOSU with lower back against the dome.
3. Head and gaze forward.
4. Reach both arms forward, palms down, slightly above shoulder height.
5. Knees bent. Feet on the mat, slightly apart.

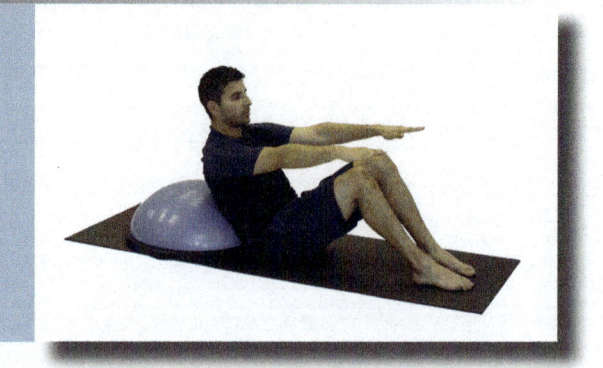

Exercise

Inhale   To prepare.

Exhale   Deepen the curl forward, while maintaining the lower back connection with the dome.

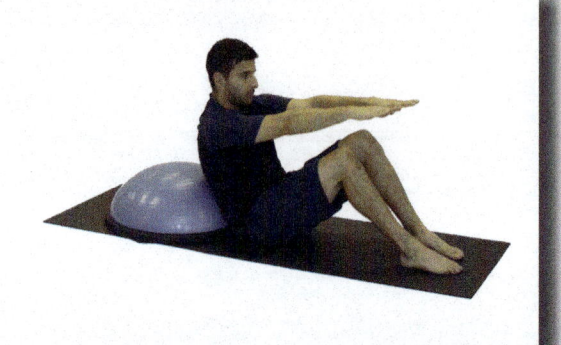

Inhale   Lift and suspend both legs to tabletop.

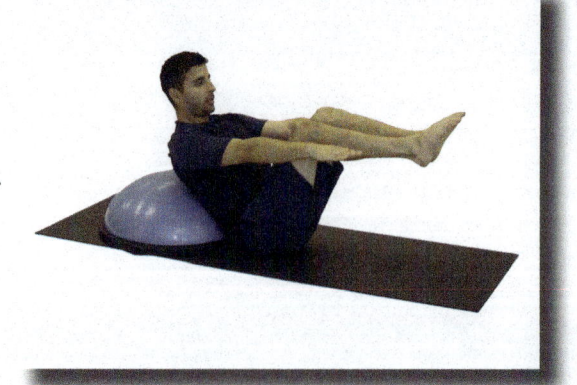

Exhale   Lower R foot to the mat keeping L knee and foot in tabletop.

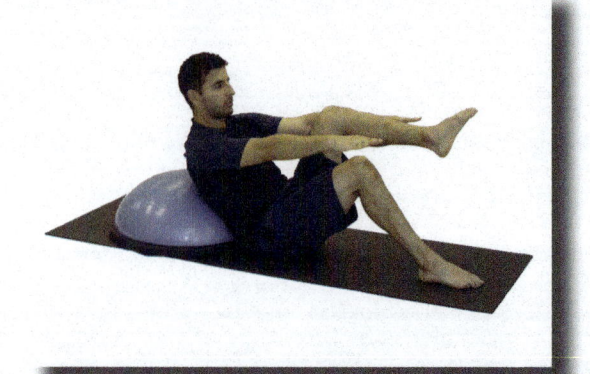

84   **EXERCISES**

Inhale   Lift R leg back to tabletop.

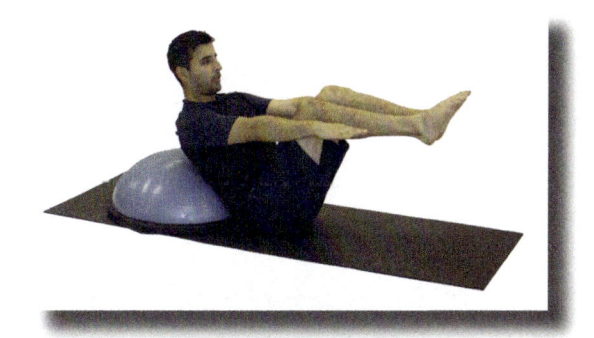

Exhale   Lower L foot back to the mat, keeping R knee and foot in tabletop.

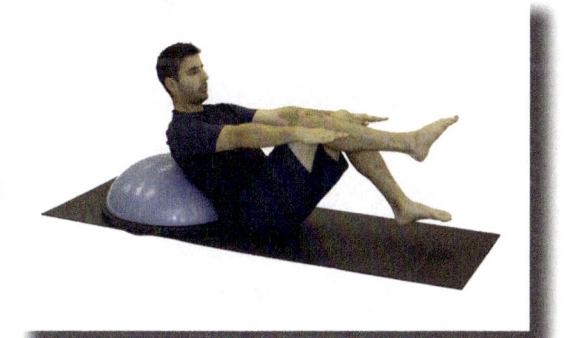

Inhale   Bring L foot back to tabletop.
Reps   X5-10 Sets
Inhale   Return to **Start Position**.

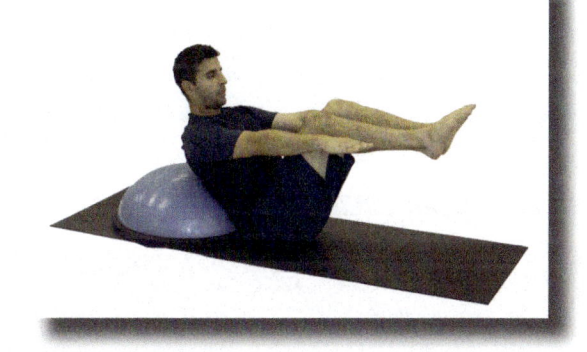

Modified
1. Sitting on the dome, lift one leg only - stay in the curl. Reps X5-10 Sets (SIMPLIFY)

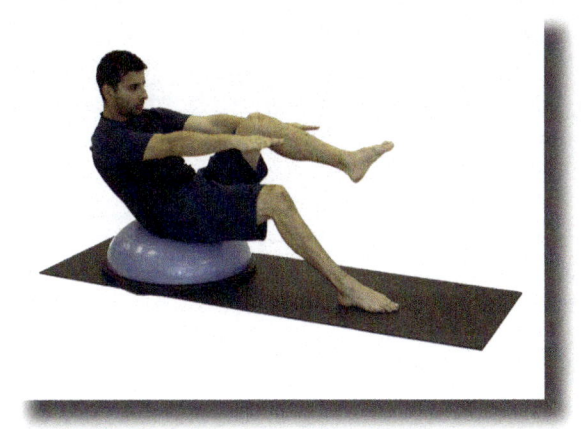

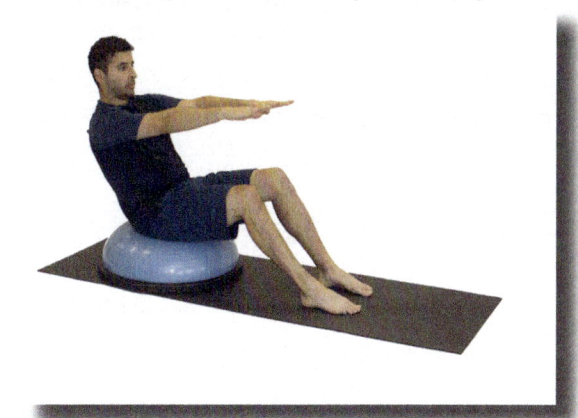

FUNDAMENTALS   85

2. Sit on the dome, lift and lower both legs without suspending. Hold the back of knees. Reps X5-10 (CHALLENGE)

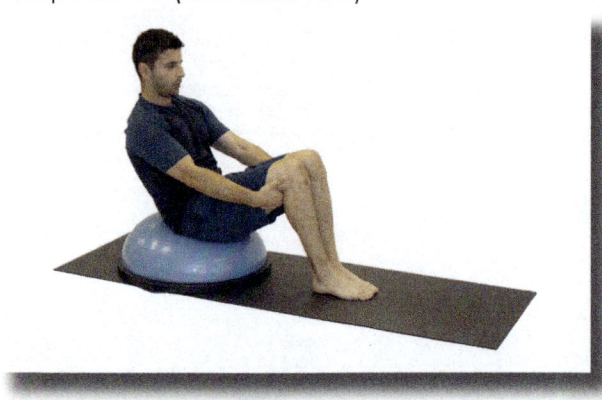

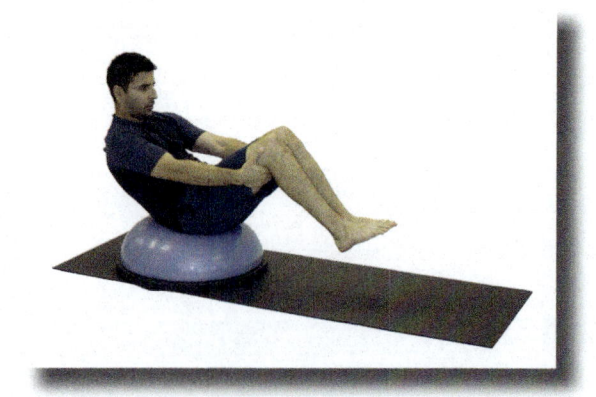

3. Sitting on the floor in front of the BOSU, lift and suspend, then lower both legs. Keep arms reaching forward. Reps X5-10 (CHALLENGE)

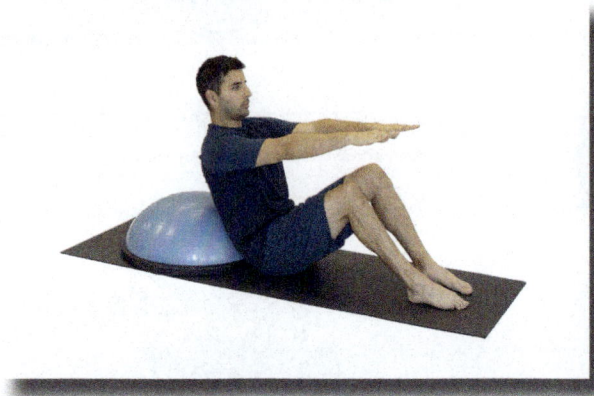

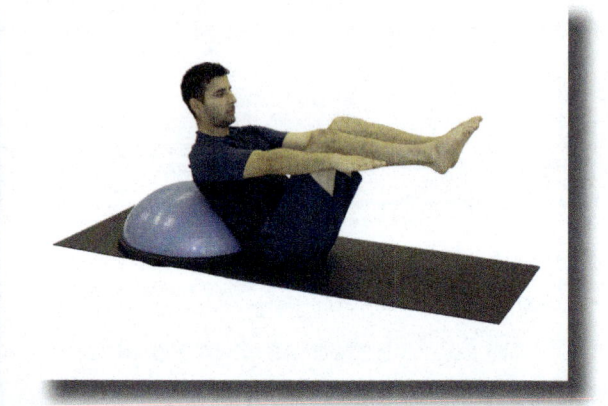

Muscular Intention

- Stabilizing the pelvis using the deep abdominals.
- Maintaining scapular depression using scapular stabilizers.

Tips

- ✔ Slide the shoulders down the back and keep the collar bones wide.
- ✔ Deepen the abdominal connection.
- ✔ Use breath control during leg suspension.
- ✔ Control the leg switch with breath and abdominals.

(28) SIDE LYING CLAM SERIES

Start Position

1. Side lying with the R ribs on the BOSU.
2. R hip on the mat.
3. R hand supports the head.
4. L hand on L hip.
5. Knees bent at 90° stacked on top of one another.

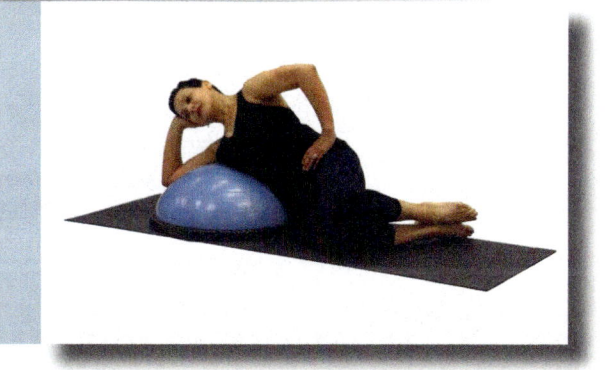

SUB-EXERCISE 1 – OPEN TOP KNEE

Inhale   To prepare.
Exhale   Lift L knee. Toes stay connected to each other.

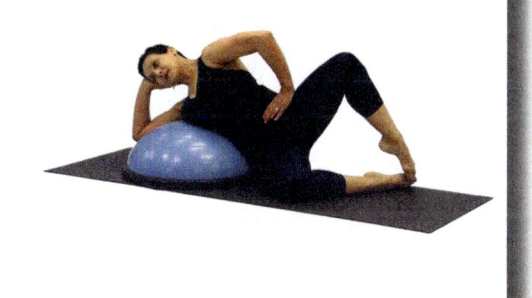

Inhale   Return to **Start Position**.
Reps   X5-10 L/R

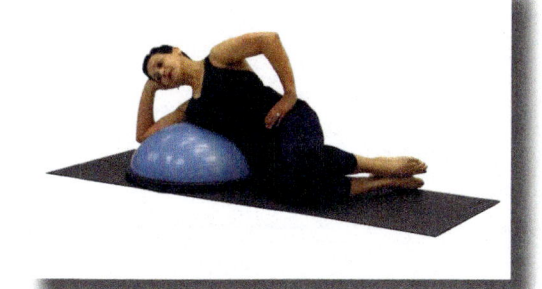

Modified

1. Lift and lower both feet. Keep the knees down. Reps X5-10 L/R (SIMPLIFY)

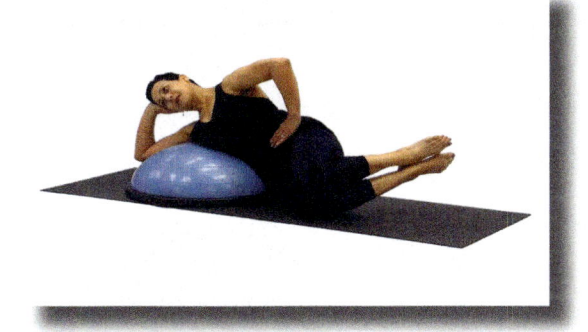

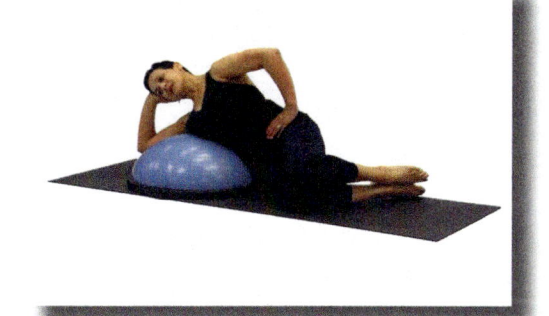

FUNDAMENTALS

2. Elevated Clam - keep the feet lifted, open and close top knee.
   Reps X5-10 L/R (CHALLENGE)

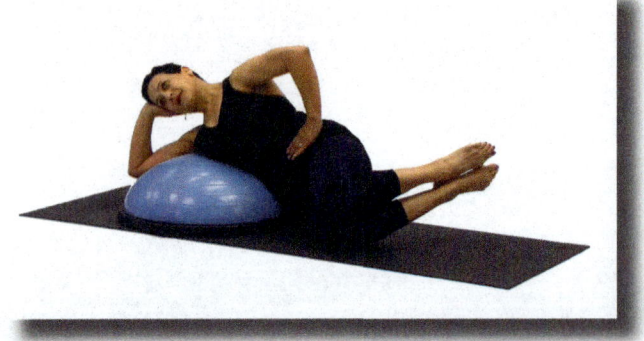

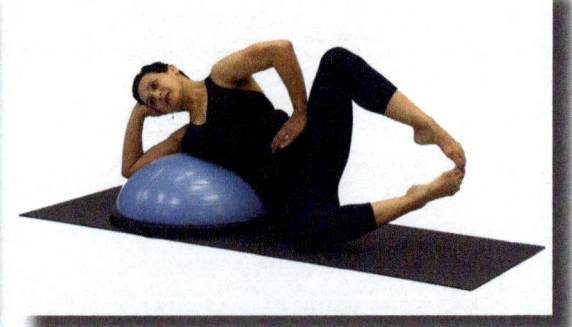

SUB-EXERCISE 2 – KNEE AND FOOT LIFT INTO EXTENSION

Inhale   Lift L knee and foot to hip height – hovering.

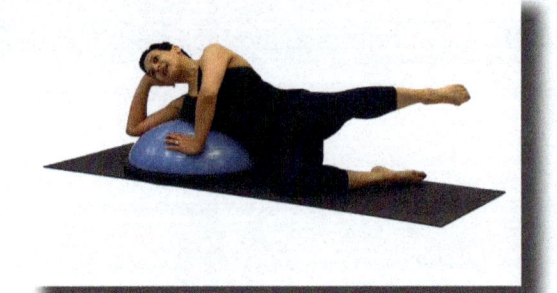

Exhale   Extend the leg to hip height, keep leg parallel and slightly above hip height.

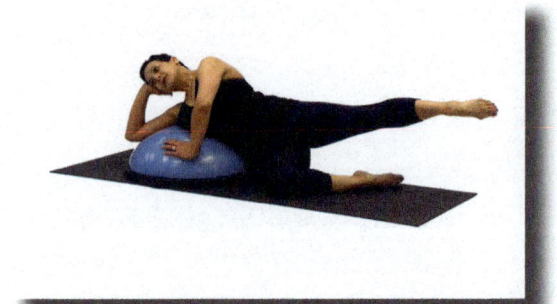

Inhale   Return to hovering.

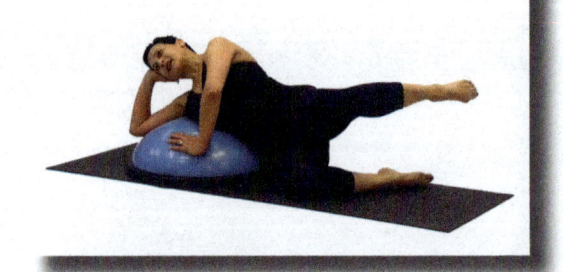

Exhale   Lower knee and foot to **Start Position**.
Reps   X5-10 L/R

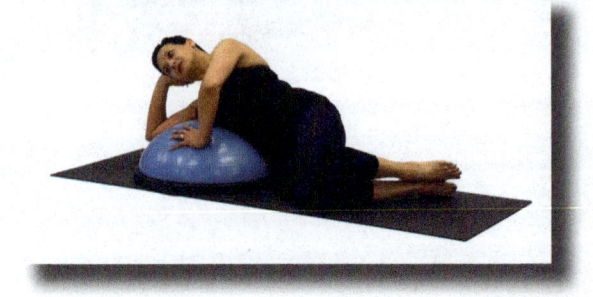

88 EXERCISES

Modified

1. Pulse the straight leg up and down. Can pulse with flexed or pointed foot. Reps X10 L/R (CHALLENGE)
2. Circle the leg at hip height and place the L hand on the dome. Reps X10 L/R (CHALLENGE)

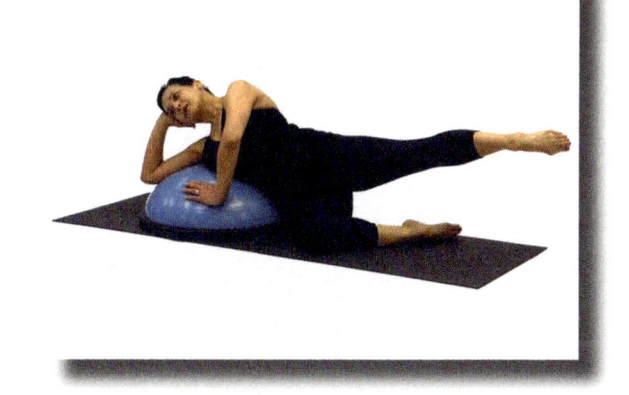

3. Point and flex the extended hovering leg. Reps X10 L/R (CHALLENGE)

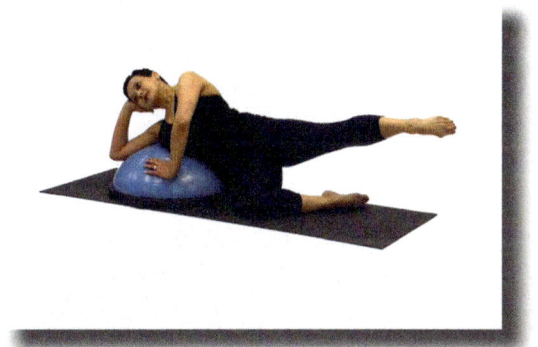

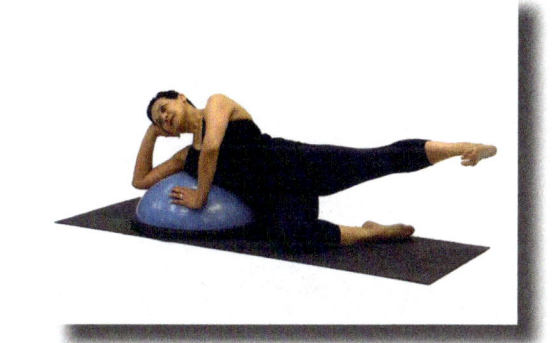

SUB-EXERCISE 3 - KNEE-TO-KNEE

Inhale   To prepare.

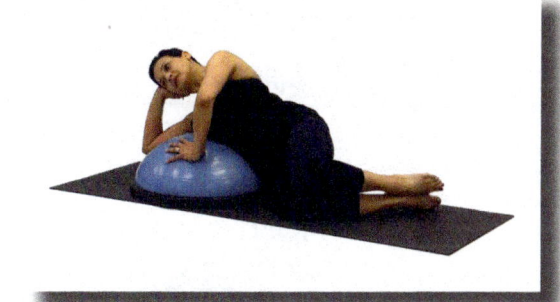

Exhale   Lift L knee and foot to hover.

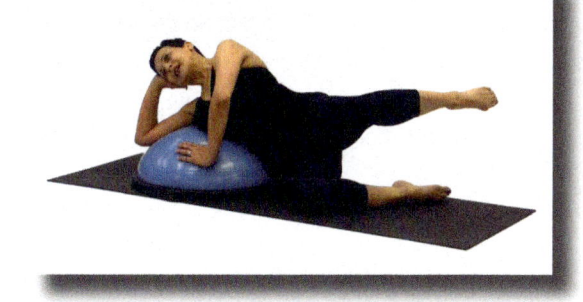

FUNDAMENTALS   89

Inhale	Internally rotate the leg and touch knee-to-knee.	
Exhale	Return to hover.	
Inhale	Return to **Start Position**.	
Reps	X5-10 L/R	

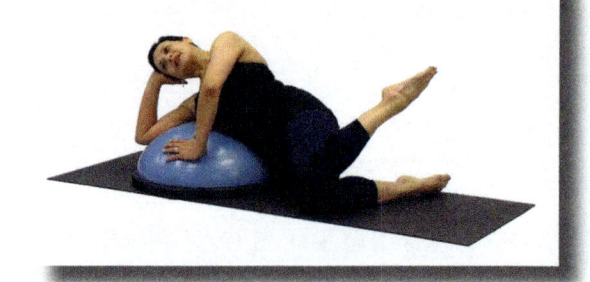

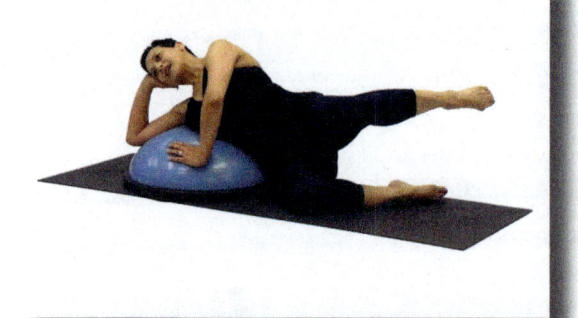

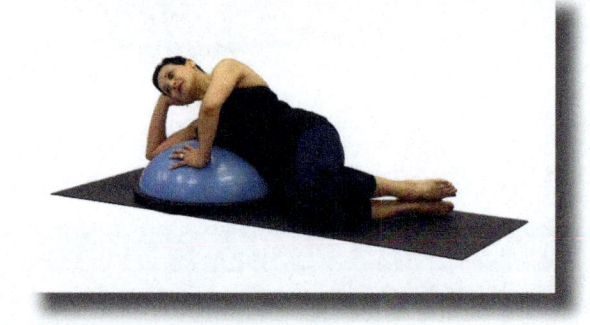

Modified

1. Pulse, knee-to-knee, keeping internal rotation. Reps X5-10 L/R (CHALLENGE)

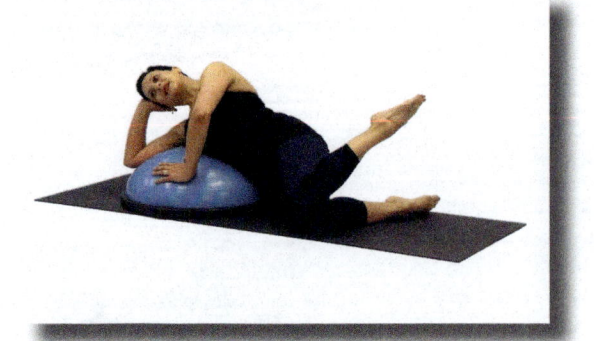

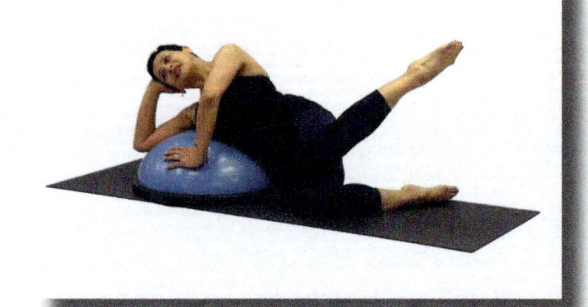

90 **EXERCISES**

SUB-EXERCISE 4 – TOE-TO-TOE

Inhale   To prepare and open L knee.

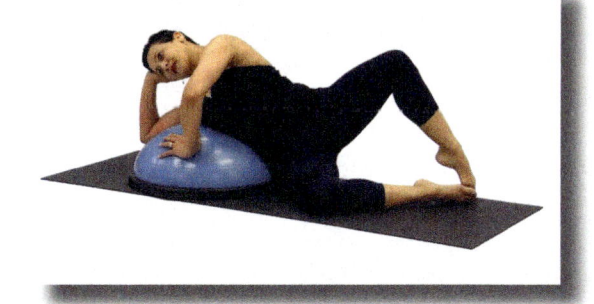

Exhale   Lift knee and foot with L knee and shin parallel to ceiling.

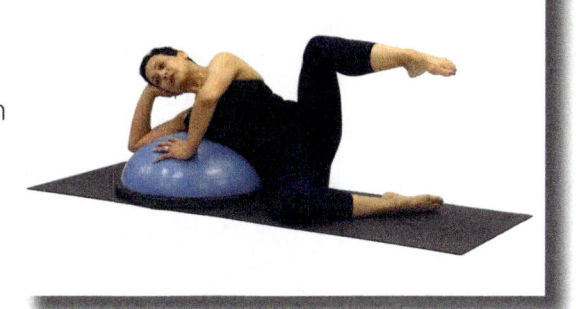

Inhale   Touch toe to toe.

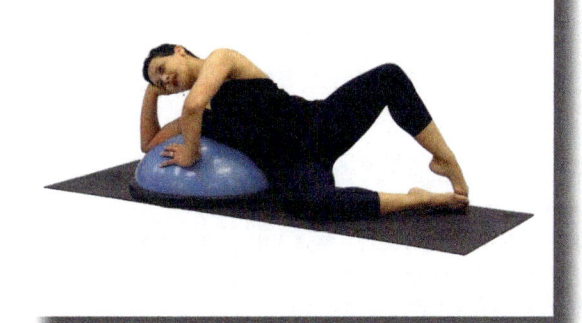

Exhale   Return shin parallel to ceiling.

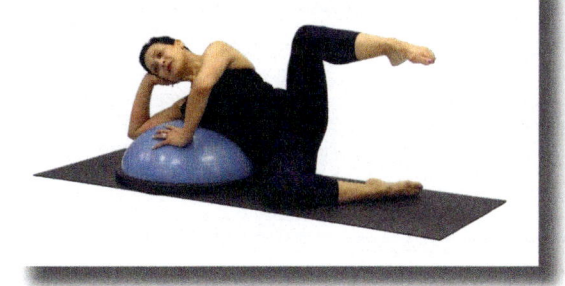

Inhale   Return to **Start Position**.
Reps   X5-10 L/R

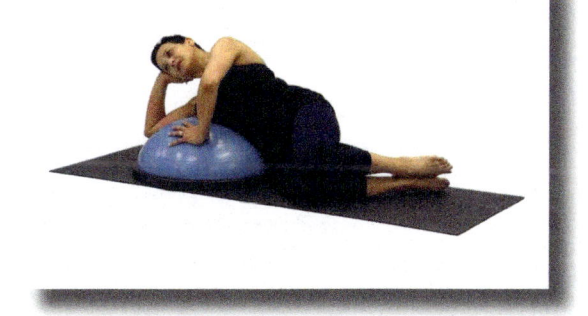

FUNDAMENTALS

Modified

1. Tap the L toes in front of the R foot and then behind the R foot, lifting the leg to tabletop in between. Reps X5-10 L/R (CHALLENGE)

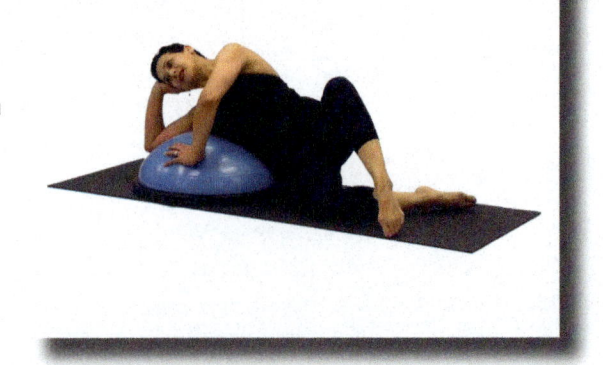

Tap in front of the R foot.

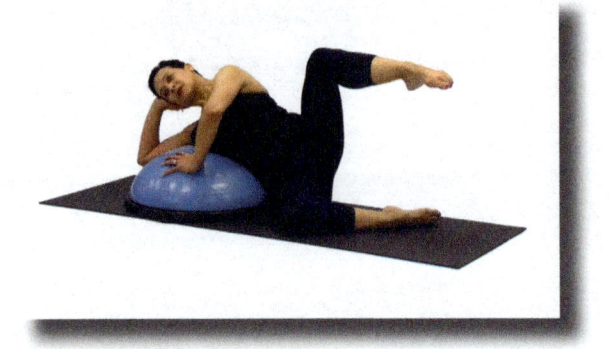

Lift L leg to tabletop.

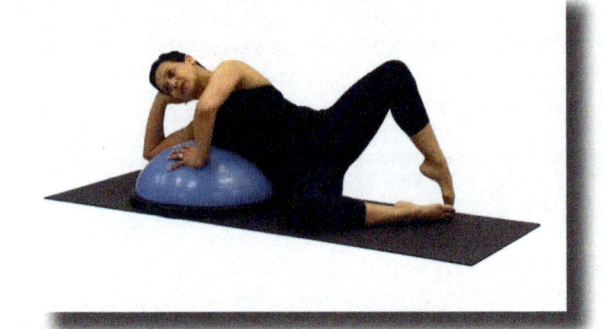

Tap behind the R foot.

SUB-EXERCISE 5 - LEG SWING WITH ROTATION

Inhale	To prepare, hug the BOSU with R arm, L hand on the dome, pushing down.
Exhale	Lift L knee and foot to hip height.

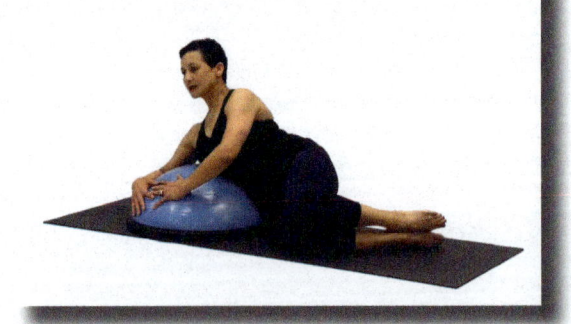

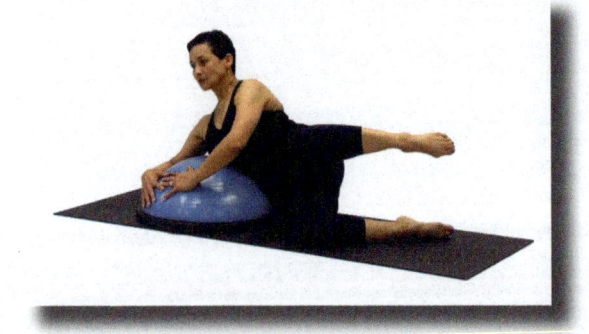

92 EXERCISES

Inhale	Swing L knee forward toward chest, look down at L knee.	

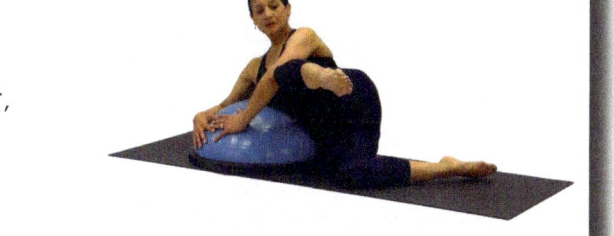

Exhale	Swing L knee away from the chest and look over the R shoulder.	
Reps	X5-10	

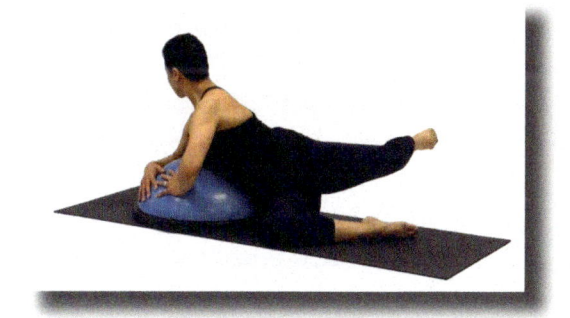

Inhale   Return to **Start Position**.

» Repeat on R leg.

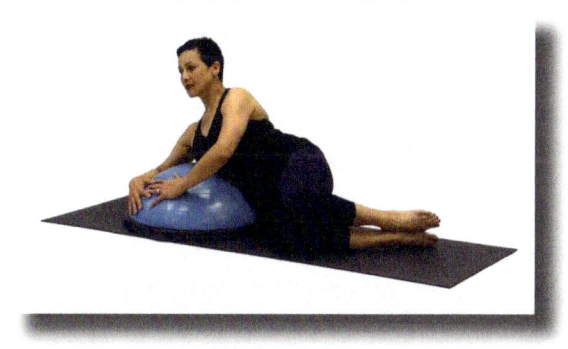

Modified

1. Pulse the top leg. Reps X5-10 L/R (CHALLENGE)

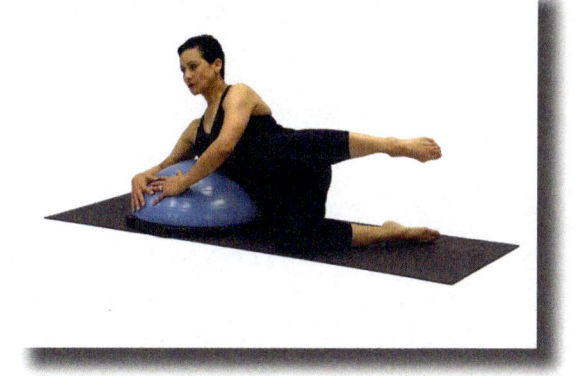

2. Pulse the top leg looking over the R shoulder. Reps X5-10 L/R (CHALLENGE)

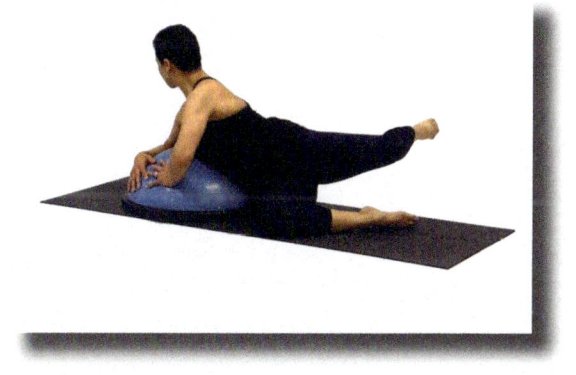

FUNDAMENTALS   93

Muscular Intention

- Engaging the glutes and hamstrings to externally rotate the hips.
- Stabilizing the torso by connecting the obliques and paraspinals.
- Connecting the transverse abdominus and multifidi keeps the hips stacked.
- Maintaining scapular depression using scapular stabilizers.
- Strengthening the plantar and dorsi flexors of the feet.

Tips

✔ Maintain neck length while supporting the head.
✔ Keep the knees and hips stacked.
✔ Press the top hand into the dome to support the upper torso.
✔ As the leg swings forward and back, keep the spine long.

(29) SIDE LEG LIFT SERIES

Start Position

1. Neutral spine.
1. Side lying on R side with hips on the dome.
2. R elbow and forearm on mat head in line with spine, looking down.
3. Place the top hand on the hip.
4. Both legs together and extended.
5. Feet flexed.

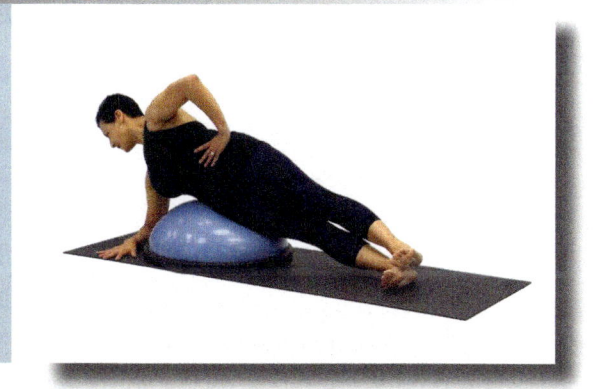

SUB-EXERCISE 1 - KEY

Inhale   Extend and lift L leg, pointing L foot.

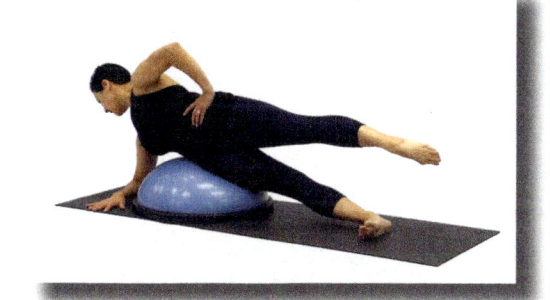

Exhale   Laterally rotate L leg (to unlock).

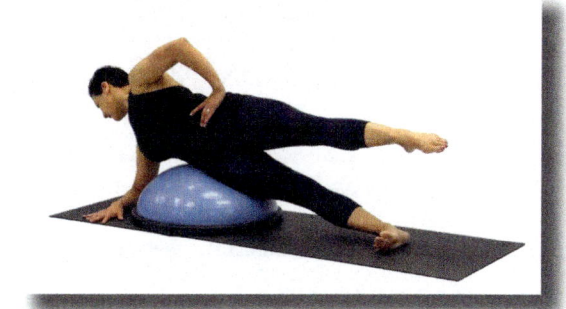

Inhale   Return leg back to parallel. (lock)

Reps   X10

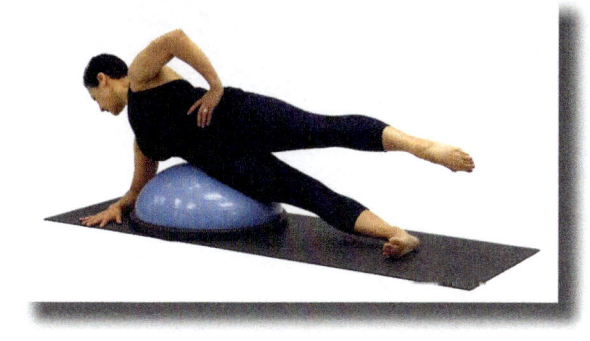

FUNDAMENTALS

Modified

1. Turn out the top leg. Return to parallel. Top hand on the top hip or the dome. Bend the bottom knee. Reps X5-10 L/R (SIMPLIFY)

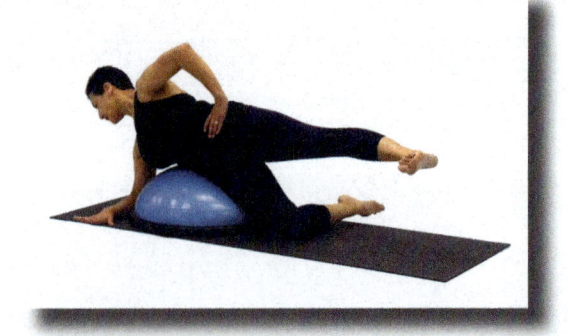

2. Keep the top foot flexed and tap behind the bottom leg and slightly rotate the upper body. Then tap in front of the bottom leg. Reps X5-10 L/R (CHALLENGE)

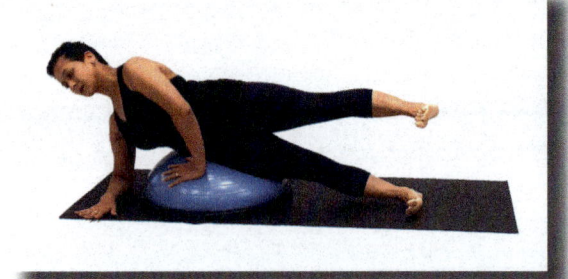

Lift the L leg.

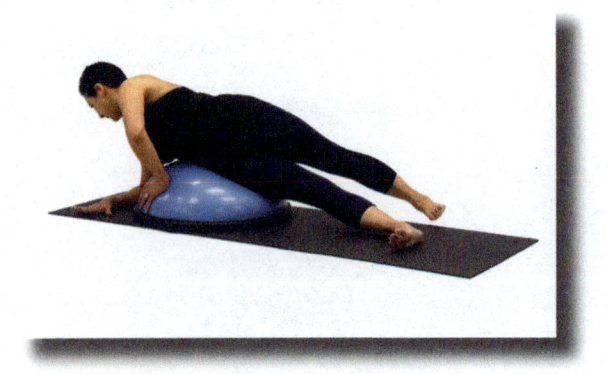

Tap behind the R leg.

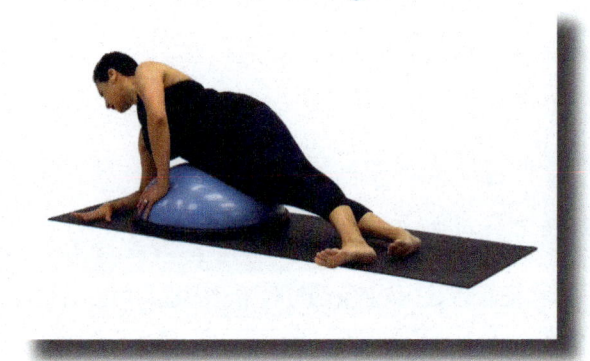

Tap in front of the R leg.

96 **EXERCISES**

SUB-EXERCISE 2 - POINT UP FLEX DOWN (BEND BOTTOM LEG)

Inhale   Extend the L leg, foot pointed. Lift the L leg to hip height (paint the wall on the way up, with the big toe).

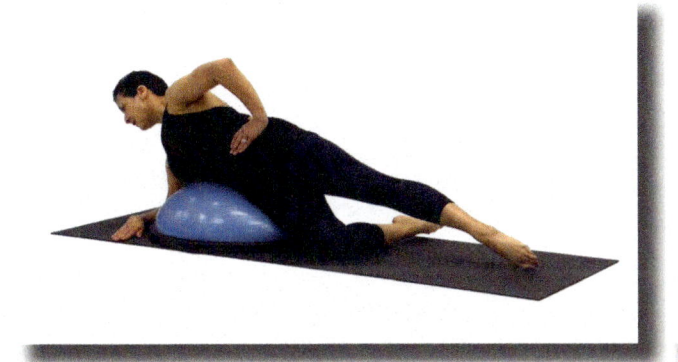

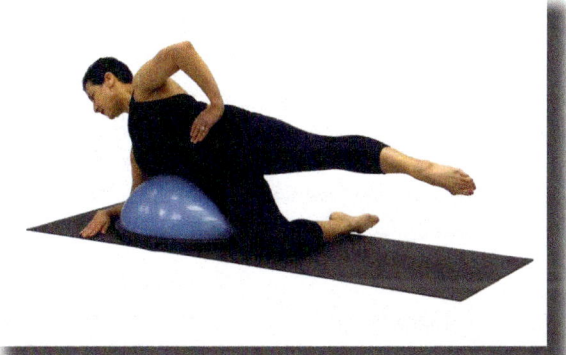

Exhale   Flex the L foot and lower the L leg, (wipe down the wall with your heel).

Reps   X10

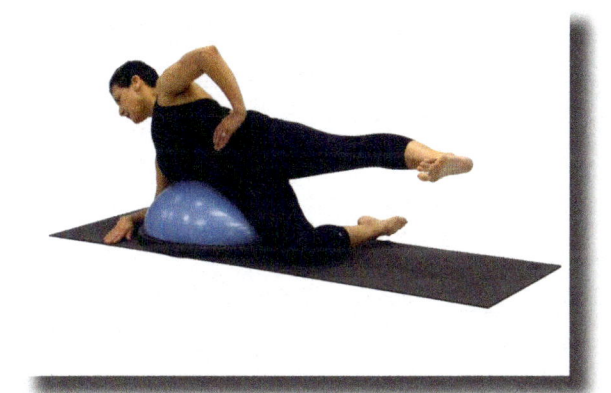

Inhale   Return to **Start Position** with foot pointed.

» Repeat using R leg.

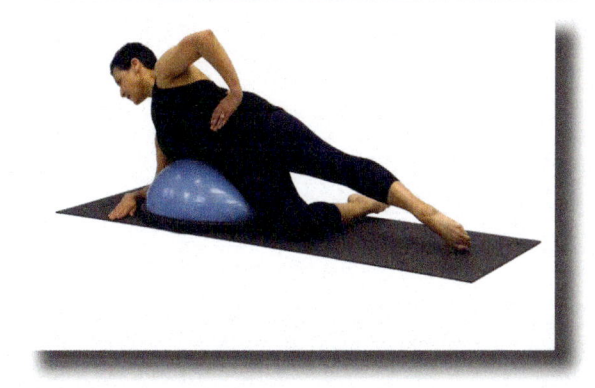

Modified

1. Circle the leg with flexed foot. Hand on the hip or on the dome.
Reps X10 L/R (CHALLENGE)

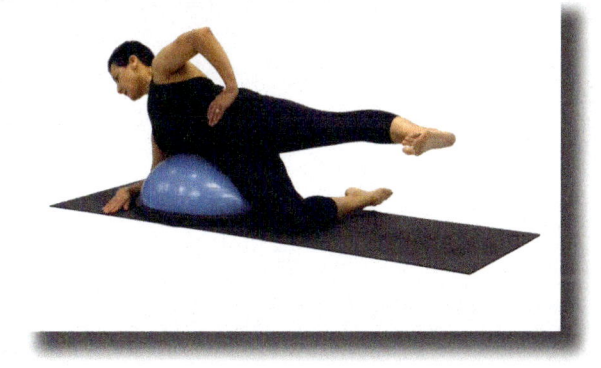

FUNDAMENTALS

Muscular Intention
- Strengthening the hip flexors, quadriceps, adductors and abductors.
- Stabilizing the hips using the transverse abdominus and multifidi.
- Stabilizing the torso using the internal and external abdominal obliques.
- Maintaining scapular depression using scapular stabilizers.

Tips
✔ Keep the hips stacked.
✔ Engage the lower abdominals.
✔ Look down at the elbow if you have any strain on the neck.
✔ Slide the shoulders down the back and keep the collar bones wide.

(30) CAT STRETCH

Start Position

1. Neutral spine.
2. Place hands and knees on top of the dome.
3. Toes touch the mat with ankles and knees together.

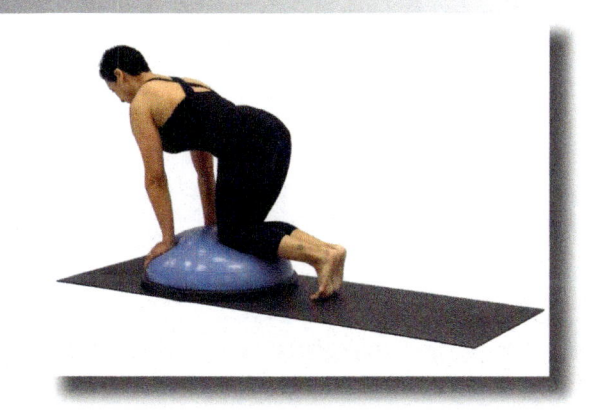

Exercise

Inhale   Lengthen to prepare.

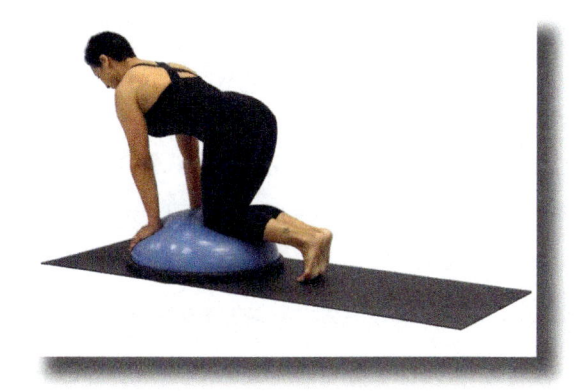

Exhale   Curl from the tailbone, the hip bones, the belly, the ribs, the chest, and ending with the head.

Inhale   Increase the flexion.

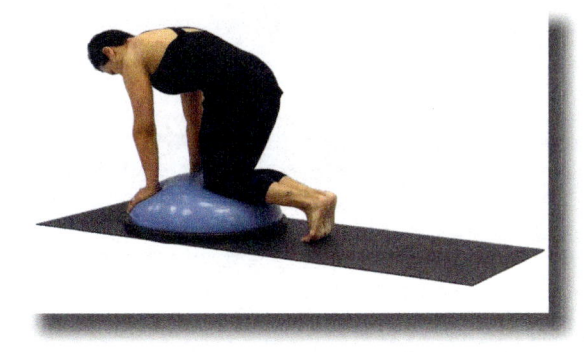

Exhale   Release spine from the tailbone, the hip bones, the belly, the ribs, the chest, and the head.

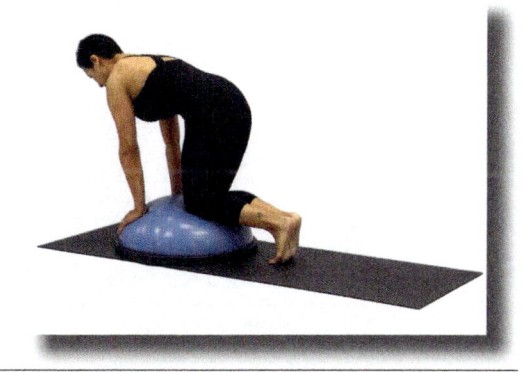

FUNDAMENTALS   99

Inhale   Return to **Start Position**.
Reps   X5

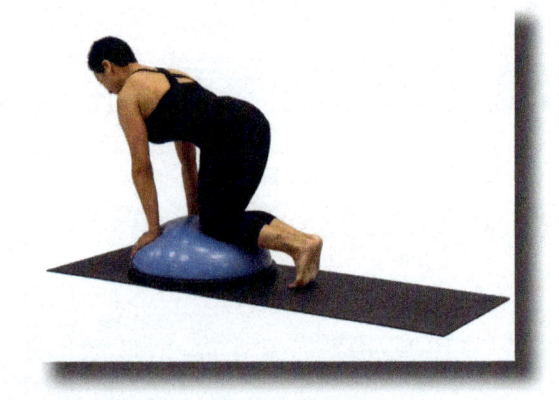

Modified

1. Knees and feet together, shins along the mat, hands on the dome. Feet pointed. Reps X5 (ASSIST)

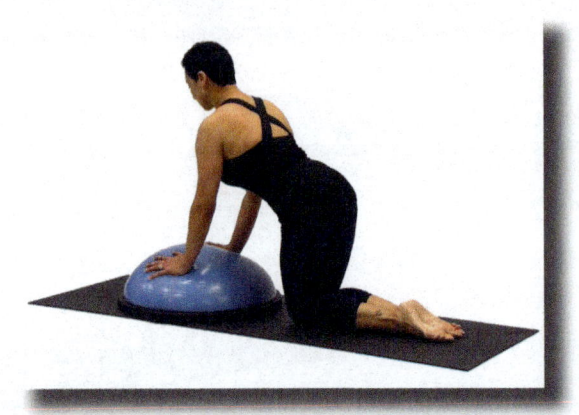

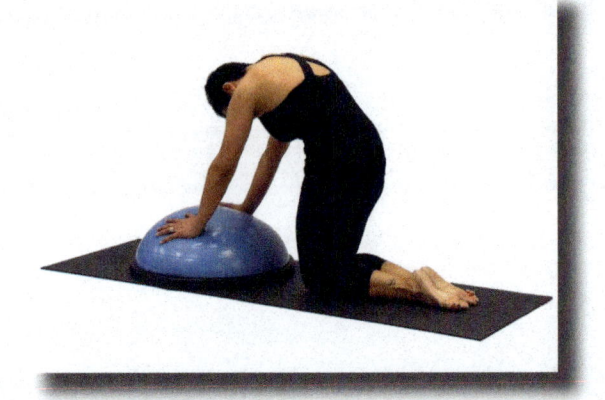

2. Knees on the dome, hands and toes on the mat. Reps X5 (ASSIST)

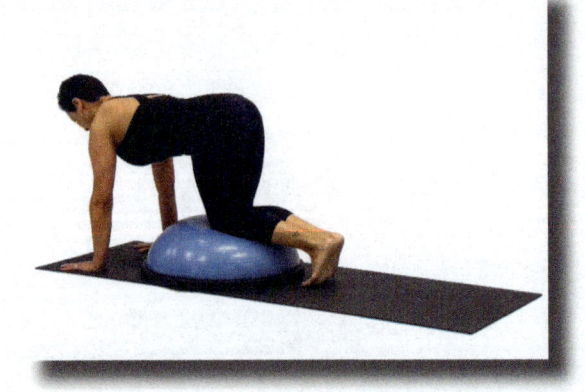

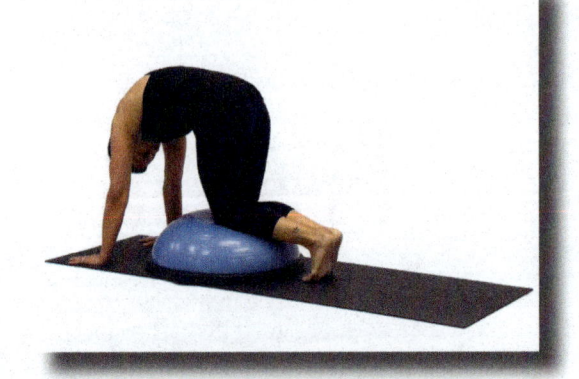

3. Place both knees and shins on the dome, hands on the mat. Shift the weight forward onto the hands. Then bring **hips** back to the heels. Reps X5 (ASSIST)

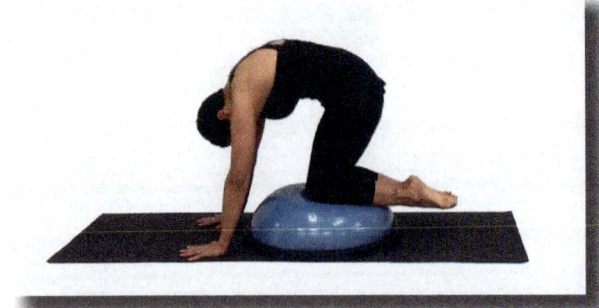

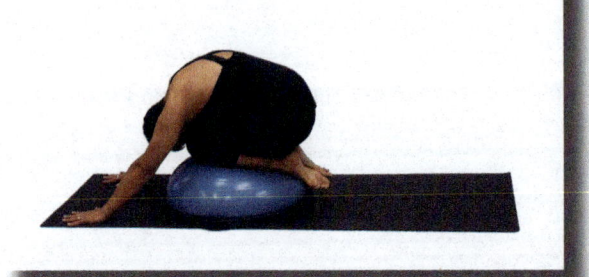

100   **EXERCISES**

4. Flat side up. Hands and knees on the dome. Toes on the mat. Keep the dome level. Reps X5 (CHALLENGE)

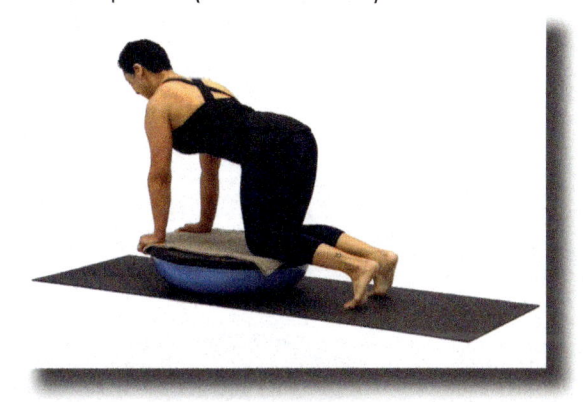

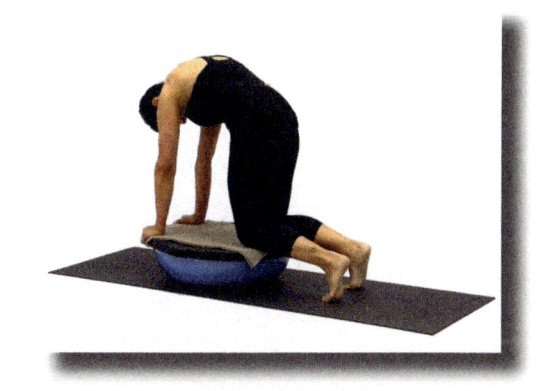

Muscular Intention

- Developing co-ordination and articulation between the upper and lower spine.
- Stretching the back extensors.
- Maintaining scapular depression using scapular stabilizers.

Tips

✔ Sequentially control the spine during curl and release.
✔ Push hands into the dome or into the floor.
✔ Increase the abdominal connection with every breath.
✔ Place a towel under the knees if uncomfortable.

(31) SITTING SPINE STRETCH FORWARD

Start Position

1. Spine neutral.
2. Sit on top of the dome.
3. Bend the knees - hip width apart.
4. Feet on the mat.
5. Arms reaching down along the sides.

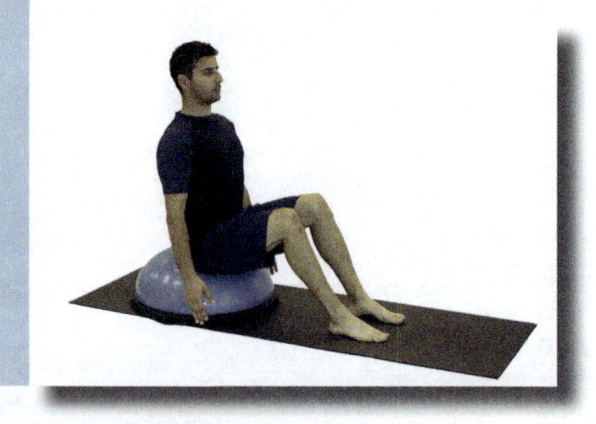

Exercise

Inhale   Lengthen the spine to prepare.

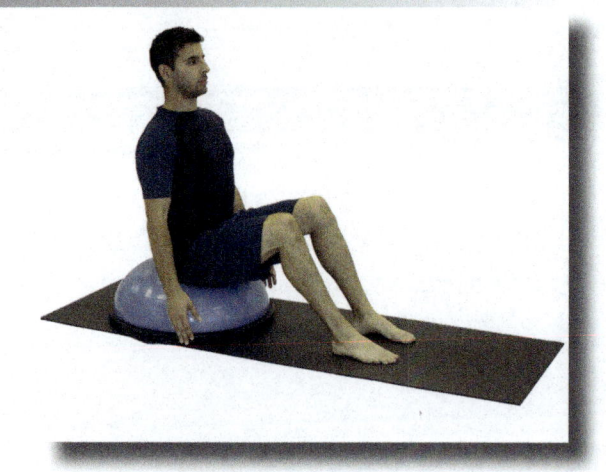

Exhale   Flex from the top of the head, through cervical spine, then upper thoracic spine, then mid-thoracic spine.

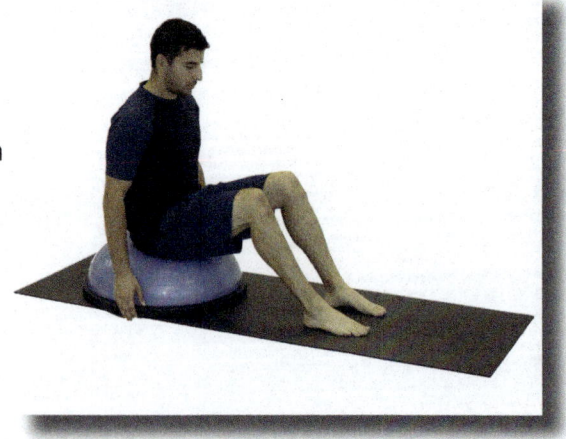

Inhale   Hold the round back position and expand the back as you reach the arms forward, past the toes.

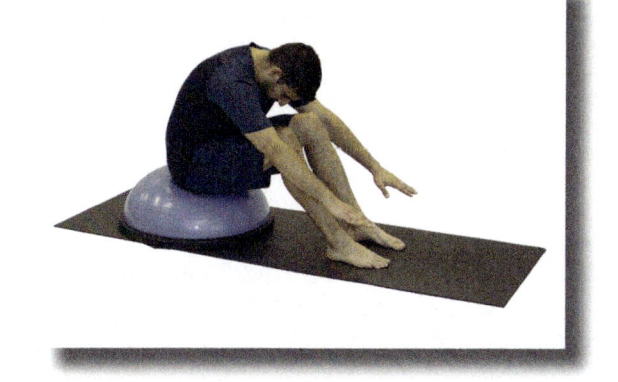

Exhale   Unfold the spine one vertebra at a time, through to the top of the head and returning to **Start Position.**

Reps   X5

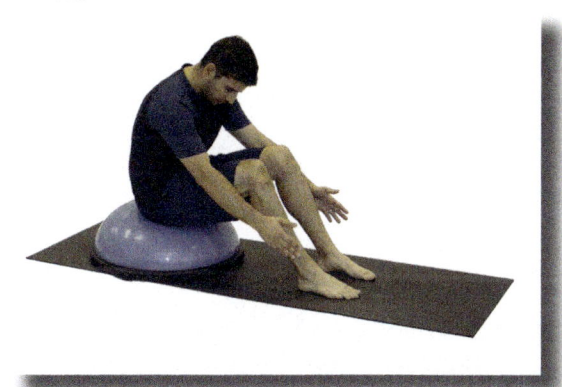

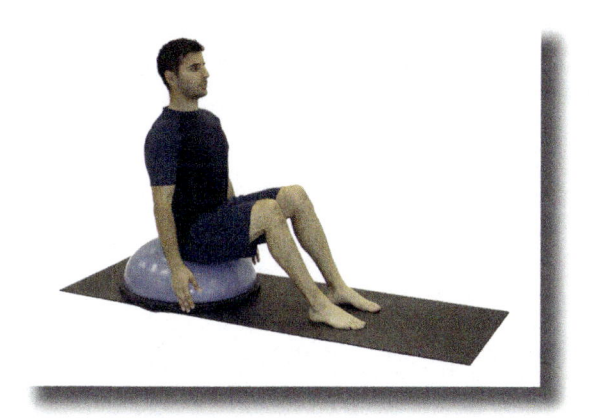

Modified

1. Straight legs wider than hip distance apart. Reps X5 (CHALLENGE)

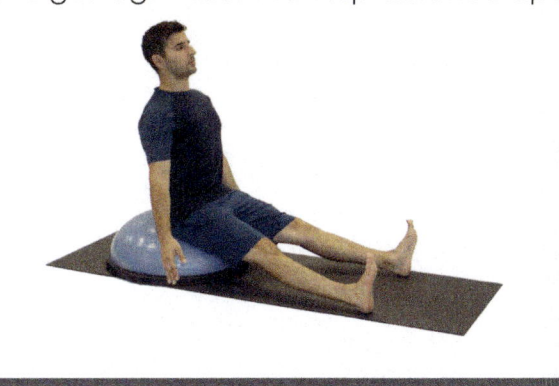

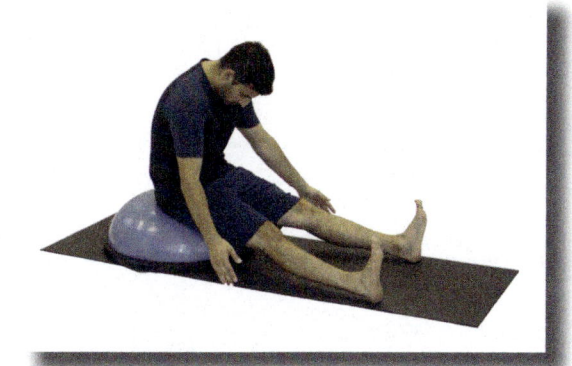

2. Flat side up. Keep the dome level as you curl forward and roll back up one vertebra at a time. Reps X5 (CHALLENGE)

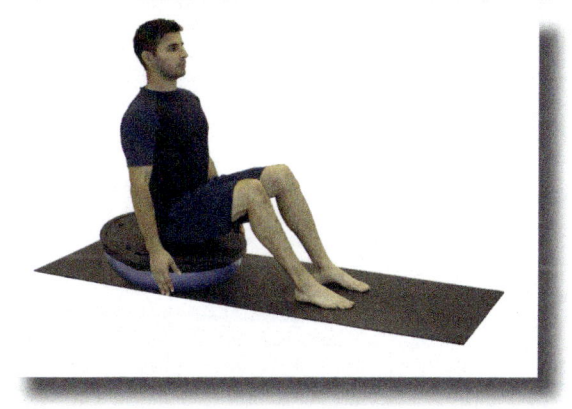

FUNDAMENTALS 103

Muscular Intention

- Stabilizing the pelvis using the abdominals.
- Flexing the thoracic spine using all abdominal muscles.
- Articulating each vertebra through the cervical, thoracic and lumbar spine.
- Stretching and lengthening the hamstrings with straight legs.

Tips

✔ Create space between each vertebra.
✔ Initiate the curl from the crown of the head.
✔ Maintain neutral pelvis.
✔ Sequentially roll through each vertebra.
✔ Stay on top of the sitting bones.

(32) SWAN DIVE PREP

Start Position

1. Pelvis imprinted.
2. Prone, belly on the dome.
3. Supporting upper body on elbows, hands in fists.
4. Legs extended and slightly apart.
5. Feet flexed with toes tucked under.
6. Head in line with the spine.

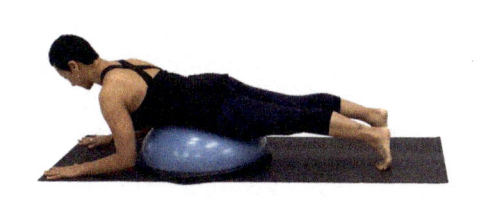

Exercise

Inhale   Lengthen the spine to prepare.
Exhale   Press the hands into the mat to extend elbows while lifting the upper torso.
Inhale   Hold torso extension.

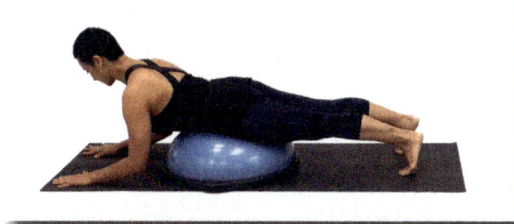

Press the hands into the mat.

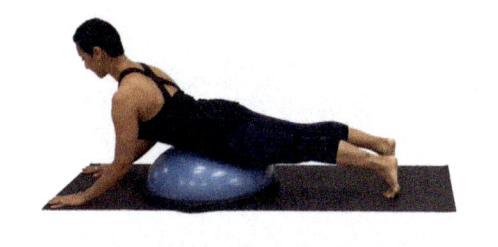

Extend the elbows.

While lifting the upper torso.

Exhale   Engage the abdominals, flex the elbows, opening the front of the chest, simultaneously lift the legs and point the feet.

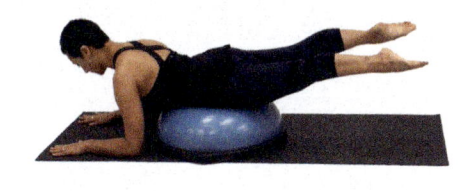

Inhale   Lower the legs, flexing the feet while lifting the front of the chest, extending the elbows.

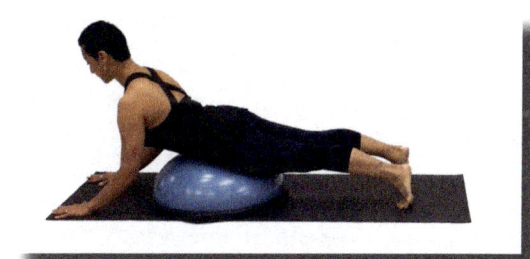

FUNDAMENTALS   105

Exhale   When reps have been completed (after rocking forward and back X5). Return to **Start Position**.
Reps   X10

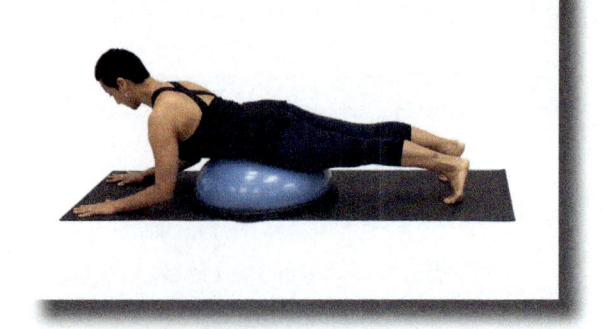

Modified

1. Keep the knees on the mat and extend the upper body only. Reps X10 (SIMPLIFY)

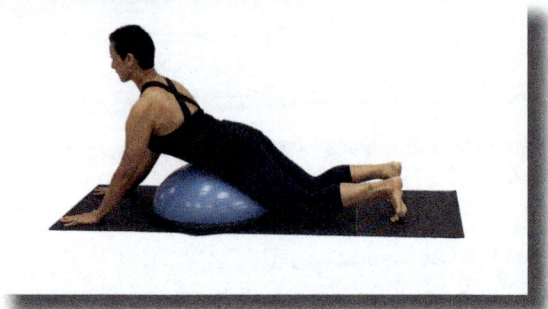

2. Lift and lower the legs only. Flex the feet on the mat, lift the legs and point the toes. Reps X10 (CHALLENGE)

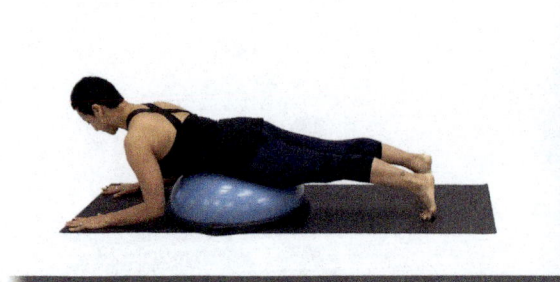

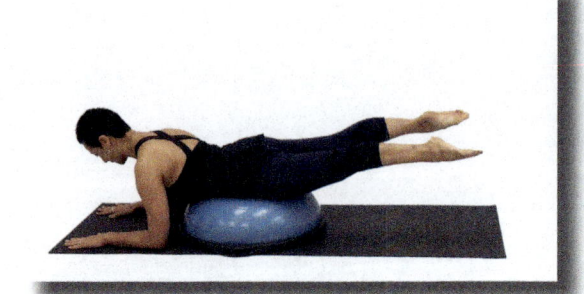

Muscular Intention

- Emphasizing mid-thoracic spine during extension.
- Lengthening of the latissimus dorsi and paraspinals.
- Maintaining scapular depression using scapular stabilizers.
- Supporting the spine using abdominals.
- Straightening the legs using the glutes and hamstrings.

Tips

✔ Engage the abdominals throughout.
✔ Lengthen the head away from the heels.
✔ Slide the shoulders down the back and keep the collar bones wide.
✔ Spread the fingers as you push the floor away.

(33) SWIMMING PREP

Start Position

1. Spine imprinted.
2. Place the belly on top of the dome.
3. Arms extended overhead.
4. Palms on the mat, spread the fingers wide.
5. Head between the arms.
6. Legs are extended, slightly apart and parallel.
7. Feet are flexed with toes tucked under, .

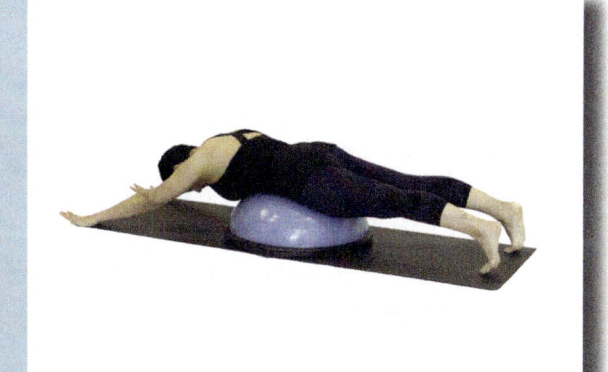

Exercise

Inhale	Activate the abdominals and lift the head and chest. Keep hands and toes on mat.	
Exhale	Lift and lengthen R arm and L leg.	
Inhale	Lower R arm and L leg.	

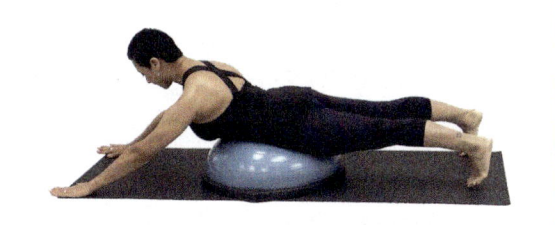

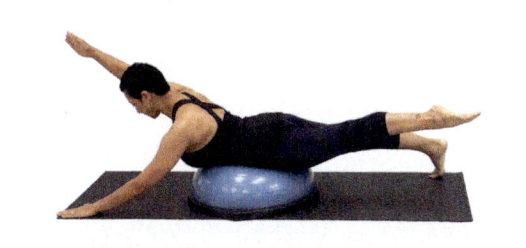

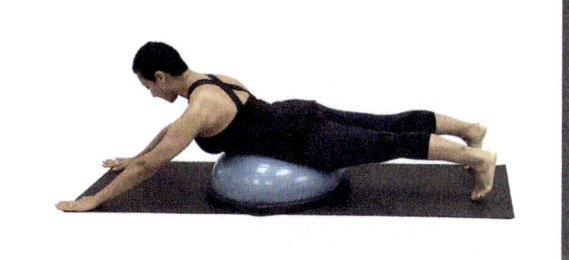

FUNDAMENTALS 107

Exhale   Lift and lengthen L arm and R leg.
Reps   X5-10

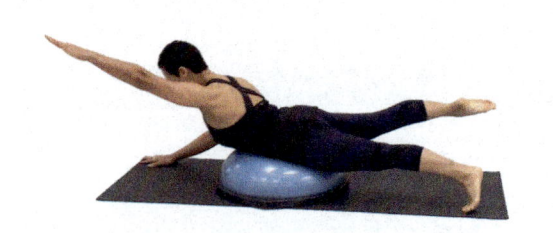

Inhale   Lower to **Start Position.**

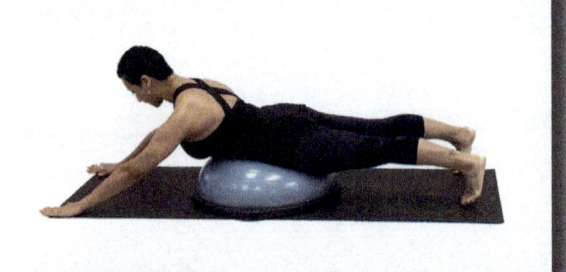

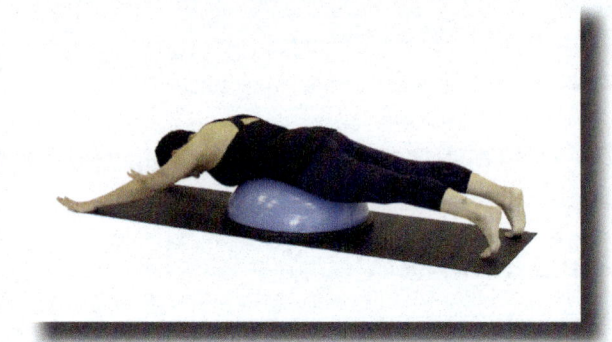

Modified

1. Single arm - alternate one arm at a time. Keep knees bent. Reps X5-10 (SIMPLIFY)

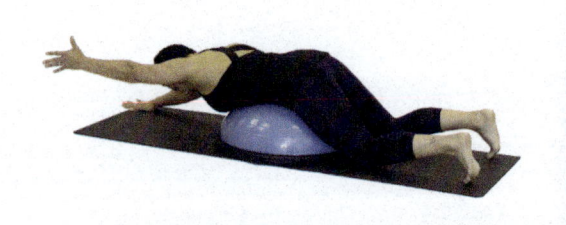

2. Lift both arms together with knees bent or straight legs. Reps X5-10 (CHALLENGE)

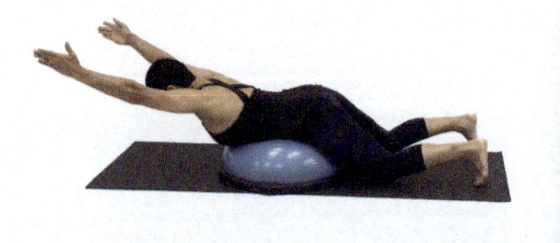

3. Lift the legs only, elbows slightly bent. Reps X5-10 (CHALLENGE)

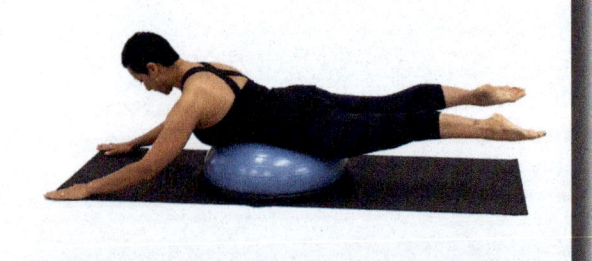

108 **EXERCISES**

4. Flat side up. Keep hands on mat. Lift the legs and point the feet, then lower the legs and flex the feet. Reps X5-10 (CHALLENGE)

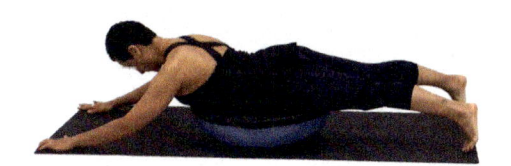

Muscular Intention

- Emphasizing the mid-thoracic spine during extension.
- Lengthening of the latissimus dorsi and paraspinals.
- Maintaining scapular depression using the scapular stabilizers.
- Supporting the spine using abdominals.
- Straightening the legs using the glutes and hamstrings.

Tips

- ✔ Engage the abdominals throughout to keep the back long.
- ✔ Lengthen the head away from the feet.
- ✔ Slide the shoulders down the back and keep the collar bones wide.
- ✔ Spread the fingers as you push the floor away.

(34) LEG PULL FRONT PREP

Start Position

1. Spine imprinted.
2. Hands on the dome, arms extended.
3. Knees on the mat.
4. Ankles and knees together.
5. Feet flexed and toes tucked under.

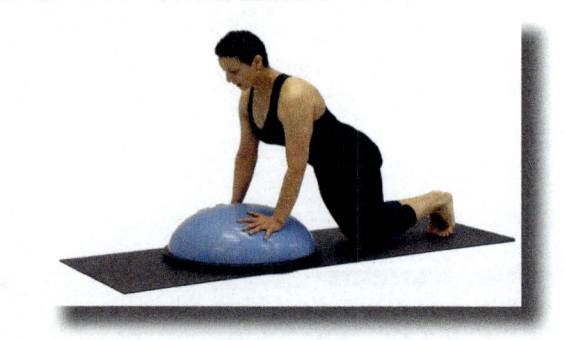

Exercise

Inhale   To engage the abdominals, lift both knees off the mat.

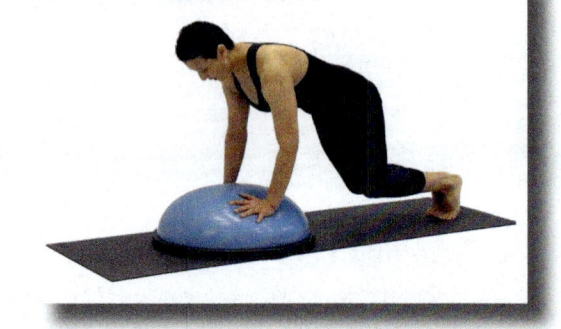

Exhale   Walk out to extended R, followed by the L leg.

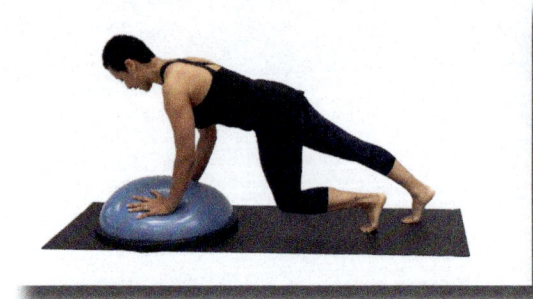

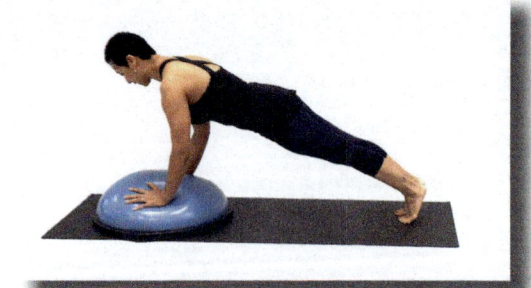

Inhale   Return legs one at a time. R knee bent and hovering then L knee bent hovering above the mat.

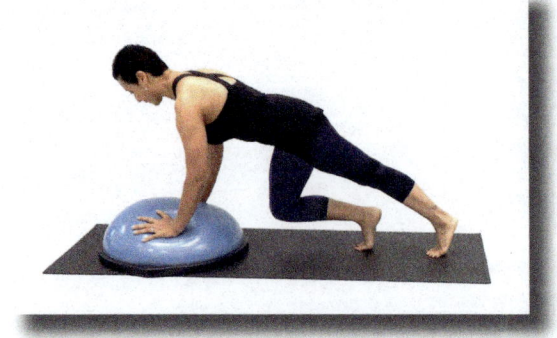

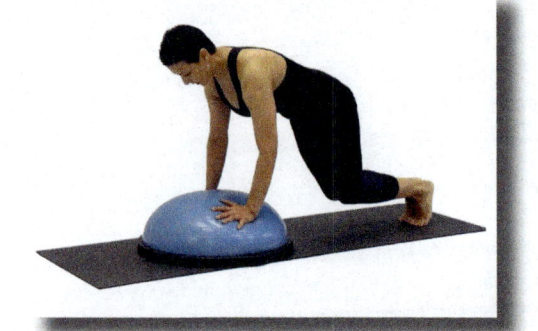

110   **EXERCISES**

Exhale   Lower knees back to **Start Position**.
Reps   X10

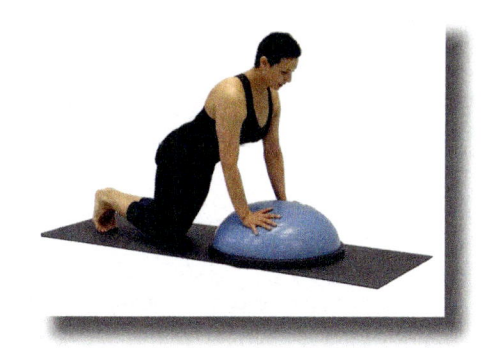

Modified

1. Place bent knees and feet further back. Lift and straighten both knees. Bend and lower both knees. Reps X10 (CHALLENGE)

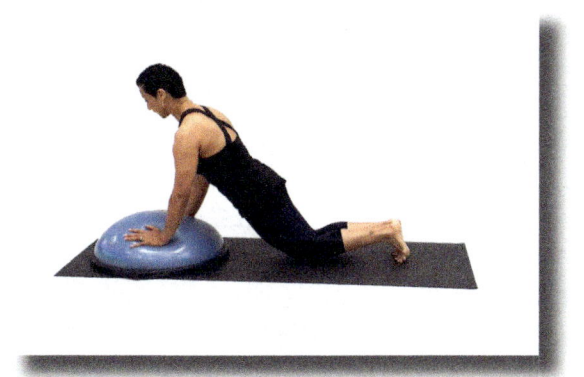

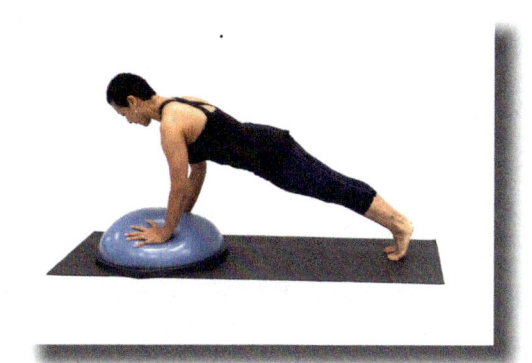

2. Flat side up, lift and lower knees on and off the mat. Reps X10 (SIMPLIFY)

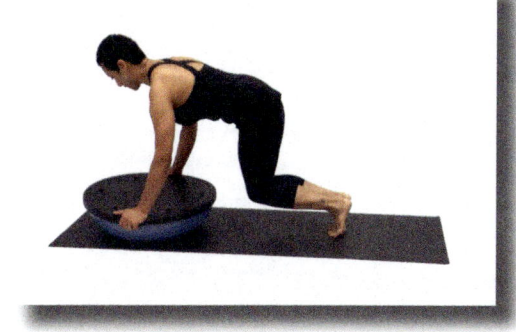

Muscular Intention

- Connecting the shoulder blades by using the latissimus dorsi, serratus (posterior and anterior).
- Stabilizing the torso using the deep abdominals and paraspinals.
- Connecting the inner thighs by working the adductors of the legs.

Tips

✔ Push hands into the dome to keep the chest lifted.
✔ Increase the abdominal connection.
✔ Slide the shoulders down the back and keep the collar bones wide.
✔ On the flat side, keep the dome level.

FUNDAMENTALS

(35) REVERSE PLANK PREP (LEG PULL)

Start Position

1. Spine imprinted.
2. Sit on mat, in front of the BOSU.
3. Hands on the dome, arms are slightly flexed.
4. Fingers pointed toward feet or out to the side.
5. Knees bent slightly apart and parallel.
6. Feet on the mat and in-line with sitting bones.
7. Eye gaze is forward.

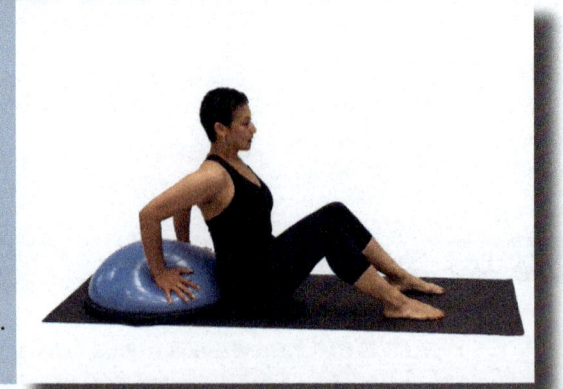

Exercise

Inhale   Lengthen the spine to prepare.

Exhale   Lift the hips upward to tabletop position.

Inhale   Hold the tabletop position.

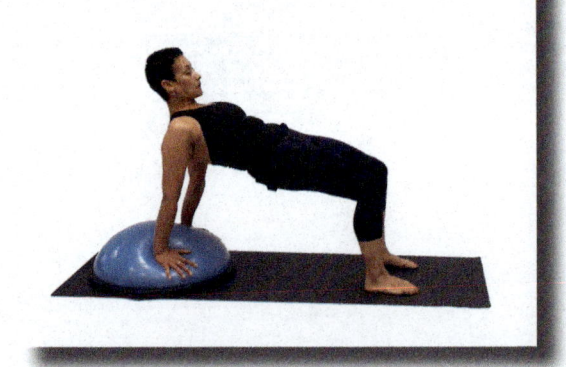

Exhale   Walk the R foot out.

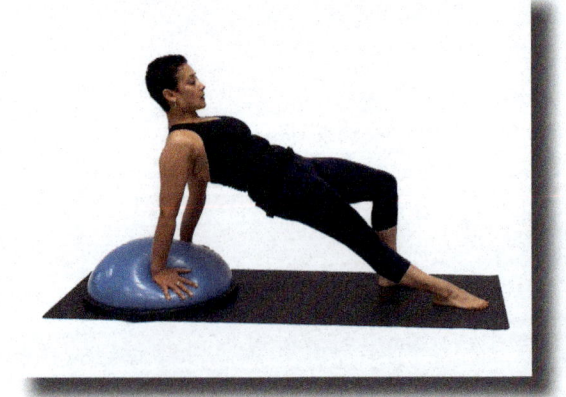

Inhale   Walk the L foot out. Legs and feet parallel.

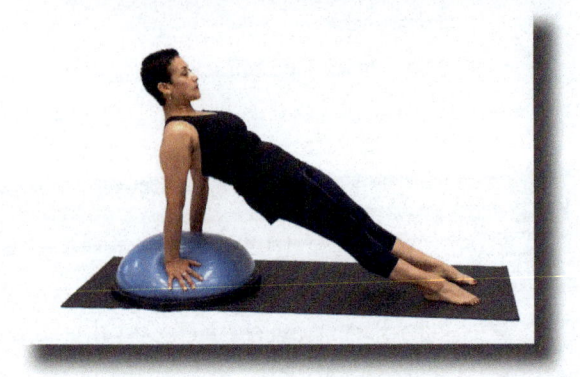

Exhale   Return the L foot.

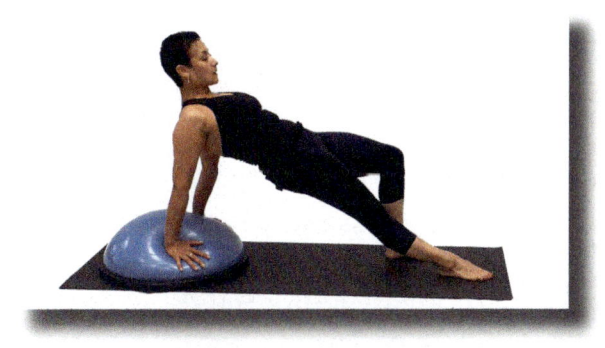

Inhale   Followed by returning R foot. Push into heels and lift hips.

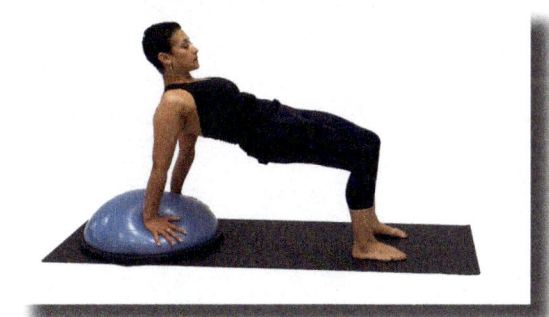

Exhale   Lower hips down to mat, returning to **Start Position.**
Reps   X5

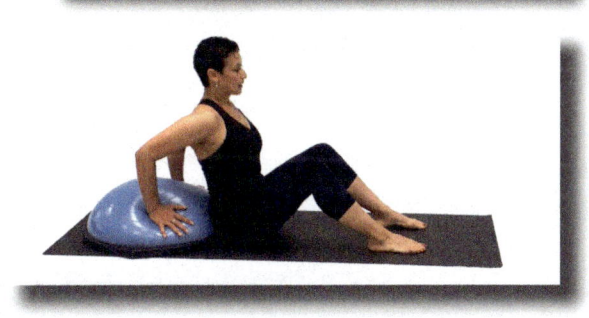

Modified

1. Triceps press hips up to tabletop with bent knees. Bring the hips down to floor.
   Reps X10 (CHALLENGE)

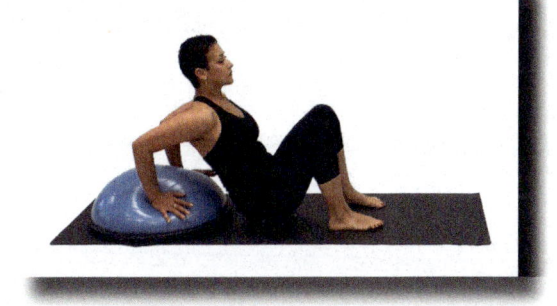

Bend the elbows, hips on the floor.

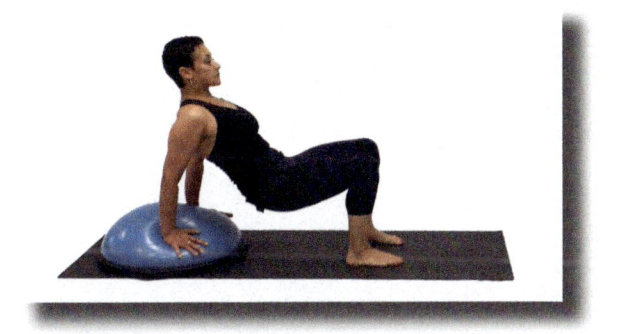

Push into both hands. Lift hips off the mat.

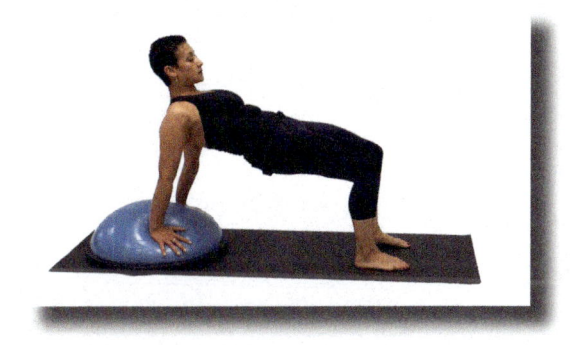

Lift hips into bridge position.

FUNDAMENTALS   113

2. Flat side up, sitting on the BOSU, hands holding the handles. Lift both hips then extend the L leg, followed by the R leg. Return one leg at a time. Lower the hips. Reps X10 (CHALLENGE)

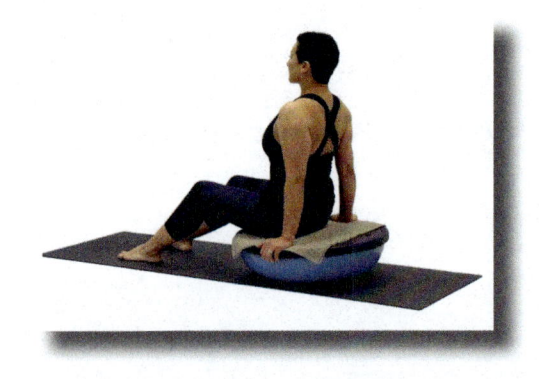

Push both hands into the dome.

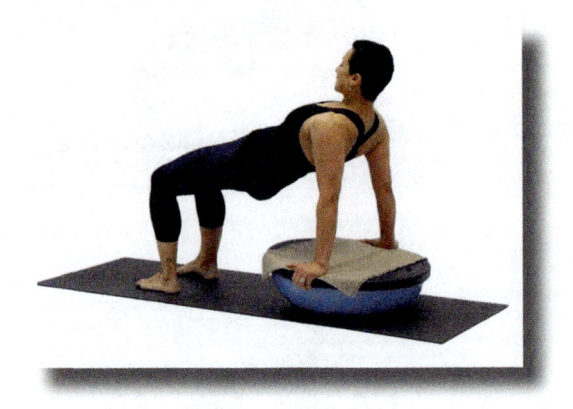

Lift the hips up into bridge position.

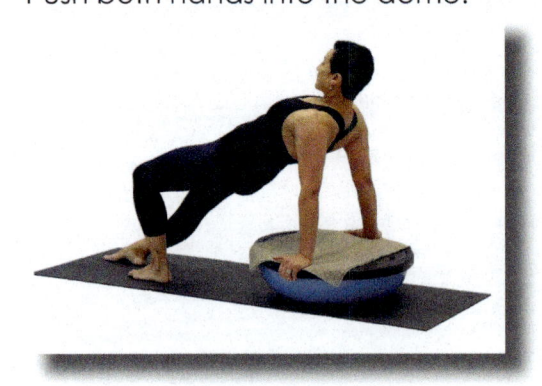

Walk one foot out a time.

Muscular Intention
- Stabilizing the hips using the hamstrings and the glutes.
- Stabilizing the torso by connecting the deep abdominals and obliques.
- Maintaining scapular depression using the scapular stabilizers.
- Strengthening the latissimus dorsi, paraspinals and triceps.

Tips
- ✔ Keep the elbows soft.
- ✔ Push the hands into the dome as you lift the hips.
- ✔ Press down into the back of the legs and feet to lift the hips.
- ✔ Look straight ahead during the exercise.

(36) PILATES PUSH-UP PREP 1

Start Position

1. Spine is neutral.
2. Hands of the dome, arms extended.
3. Knees on the mat.
4. Ankles and knees together.
5. Feet flexed and toes tucked under.
6. Hips extended.

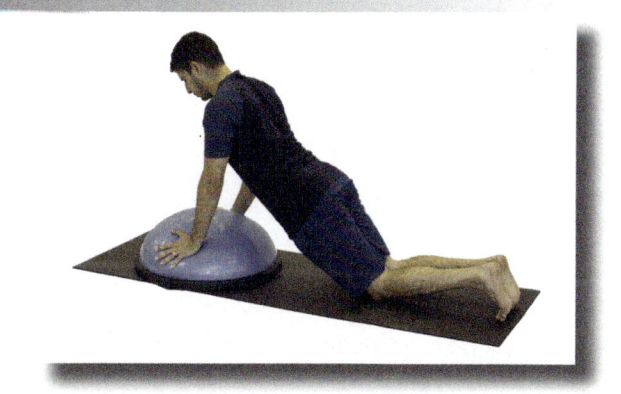

Exercise

Inhale   Flex elbows through 3 levels (high, medium, and low).

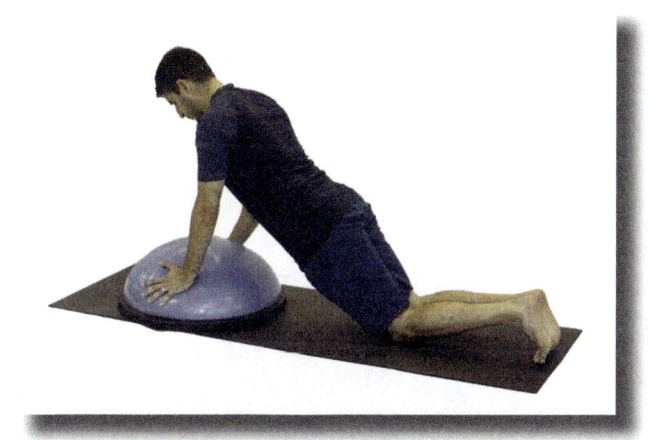

Start with arms straight.

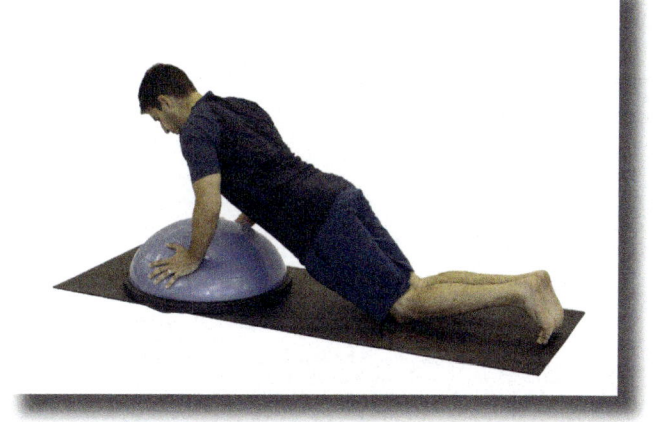

Deepen to slight bend.

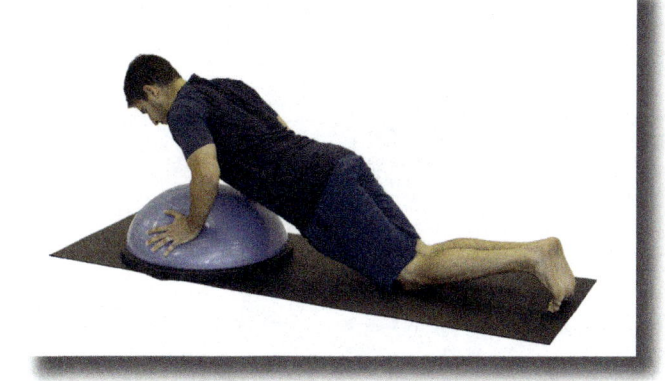

Deeper, to bend elbows more.

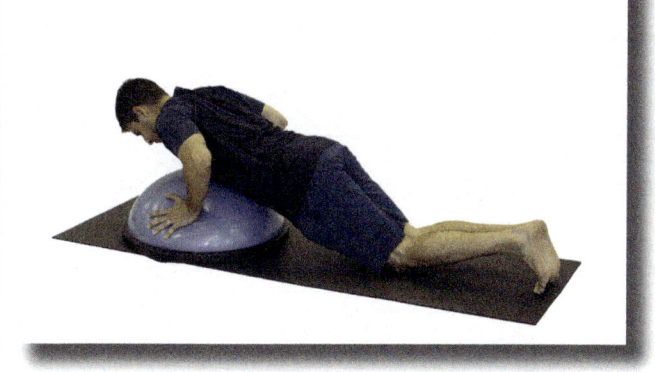

Deepest. Bend elbows as much as you can.

FUNDAMENTALS

Exhale   Push back up and return to **Start Position**.

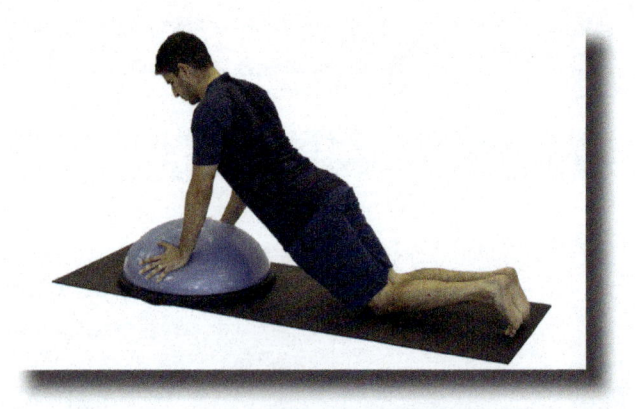

Reps   X5
To Finish...
Inhale   Push into the hands, round the back into Child's Pose.

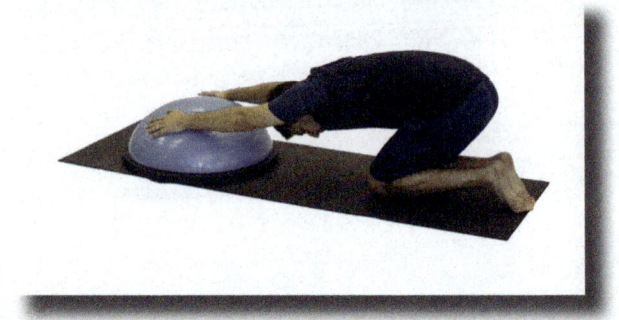

Modified

1. Hands on the mat, hips on the dome. Legs straight. Bend and straighten the arms. Reps X10 (SIMPLIFY)

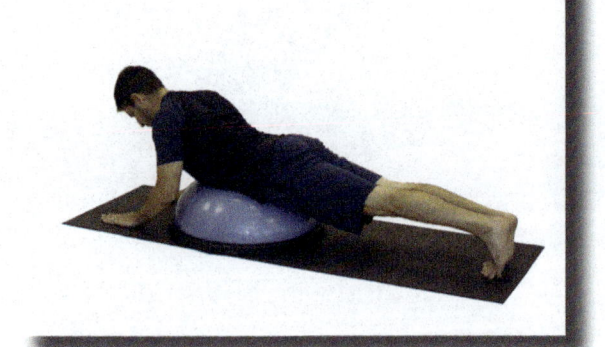

2. Hands closer together on top of the dome. Bend elbows in three stage: deep, deeper, deepest. Reps X5-10 (CHALLENGE)

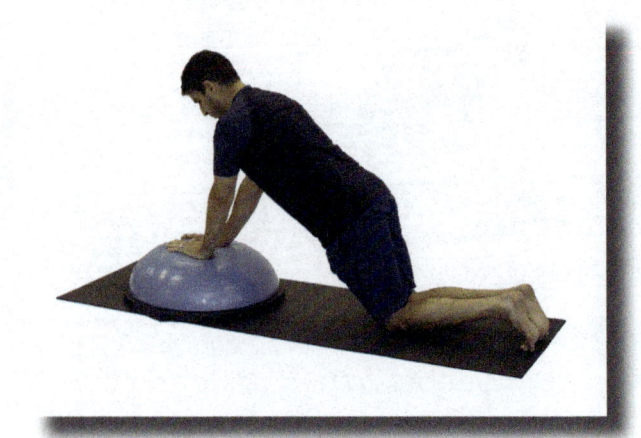

3. Extend both knees off and return knees to the mat. Reps X10 (SIMPLIFY)

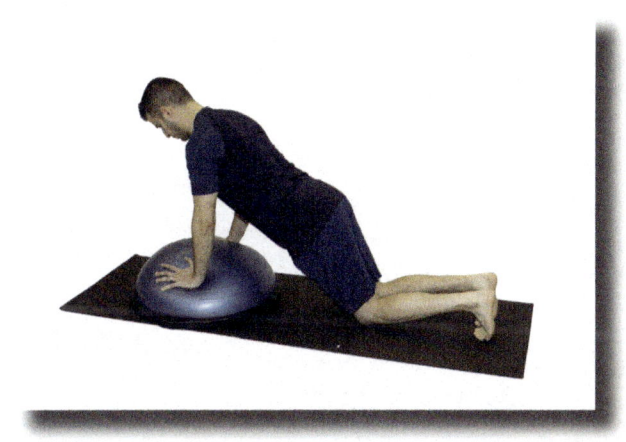

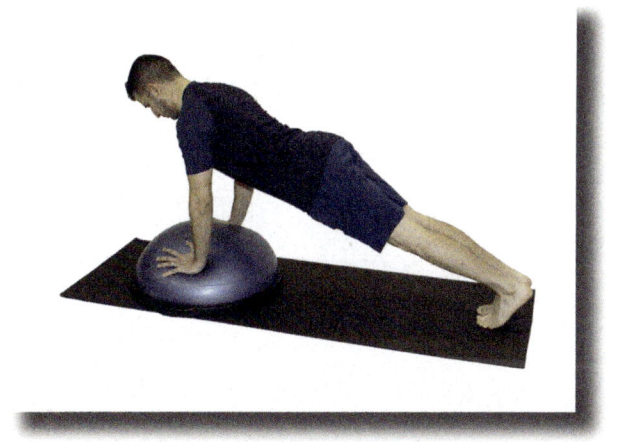

4. Flat side up. Straighten the legs then bend the knees. Reps X10 (CHALLENGE)

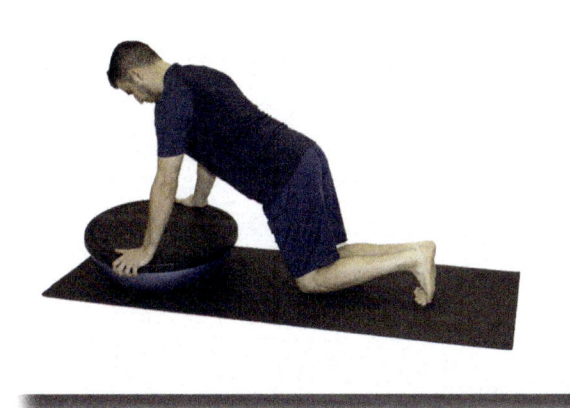

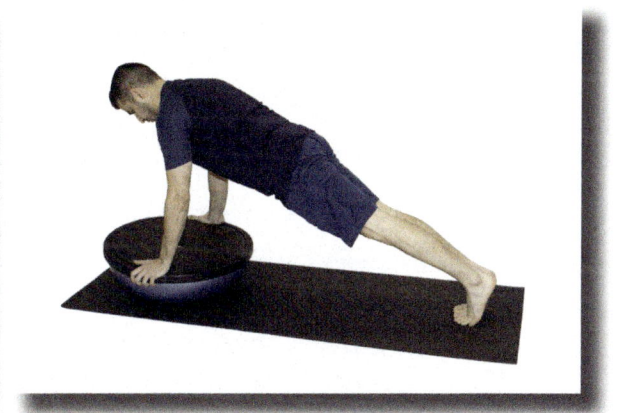

Muscular Intention

- Connecting the shoulder blades by using the latissimus dorsi, serratus (posterior and anterior).
- Stabilizing the torso using the deep abdominals and paraspinals.
- Connecting the inner thighs by working the adductors of the legs.

Tips

✔ Push hands into the dome (or into the floor).
✔ Deepen the abdominal connection throughout.
✔ Slide the shoulders down the back and keep the collar bones wide.
✔ Push the dome away from the chest with hands.
✔ Keep the head in-line with the spine.
✔ Knit the ribs toward the hips.

(37) ELBOW PLANK PREP

Start Position

1. Spine Imprinted.
2. Forearms on top of the dome.
3. Hands clasped.
4. Knees and feet together. Feet flexed.
5. Hips extended, pelvis slightly forward.

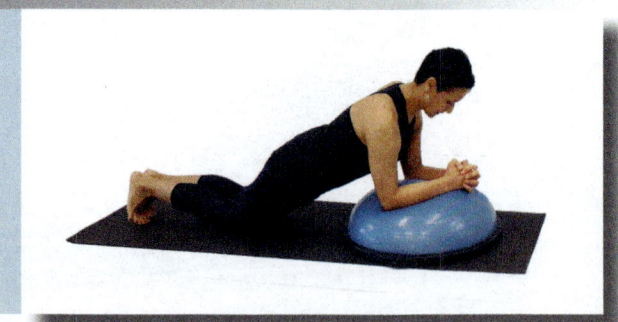

Exercise

Inhale	Engage the abdominals.
Exhale	Lift and extend both knees off the mat.
Inhale	Hold the plank position.
Exhale	Return the knees back to the mat.
Repeat	X5-10.

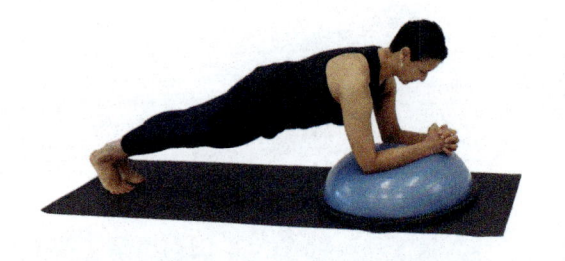

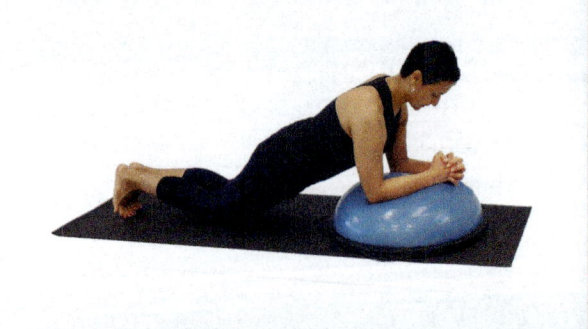

To Finish...

Inhale   With knees to the mat, sit back into Child's Pose for 5 breaths and then return to **Start Position**.

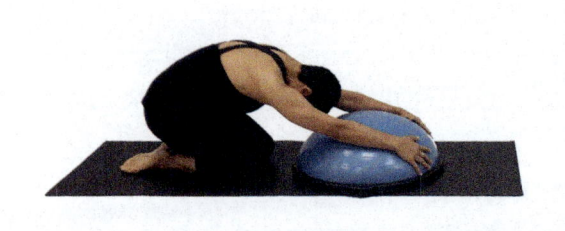

Modified

1. Elbows on the mat. hips on the dome. Feet and knees together. Straighten the legs and lift the hips and abdominals off the dome. Reps X5-10 (SIMPLIFY)

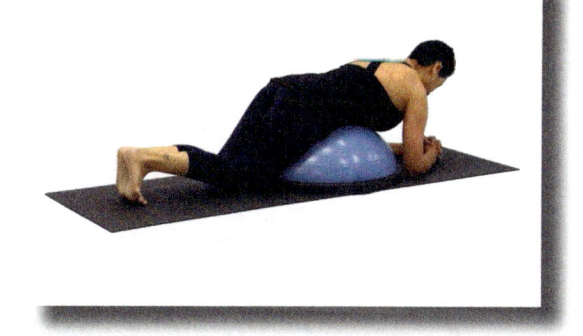

Elbows and knees on the mat.

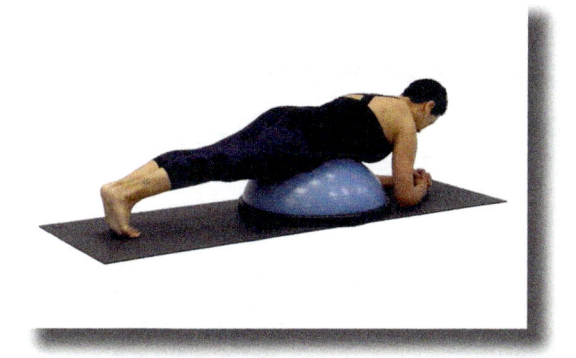

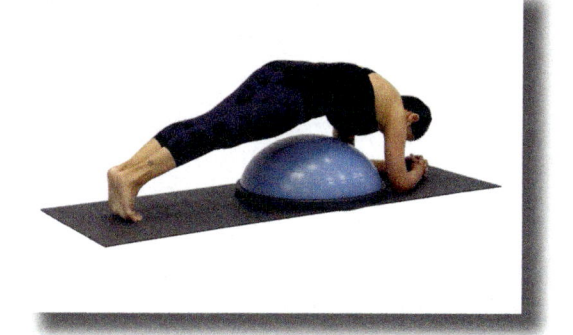

Straighten the legs.

Lift the hips and abdominals off the dome.

Muscular Intention

- Emphasizing the mid-thoracic and cervical spine during extension.
- Lengthening and strengthening the latissimus dorsi and paraspinals.
- Maintaining scapular depression using scapular stabilizers.
- Supporting the spine using abdominals.
- Straightening the legs using glutes, hamstrings and leg adductors.

Tips

✔ Engage the abdominals throughout.
✔ Lengthen the head away from the heels.
✔ Slide the shoulders down the back and keep the collar bones wide.
✔ Press the forearms into the dome (or floor) and push the dome away.
✔ Squeeze the inner thighs together.

FUNDAMENTALS

(38) SLOW DOUBLE LEG STRETCH PREP

Start Position

1. Spine imprinted.
2. Head and shoulders supported on the dome.
3. Torso along the mat.
4. Hips flexed and laterally rotated.
5. Knees bent and apart, toes together (legs forming a diamond shape).
6. Fingertips touching the knees, elbows slightly flexed.

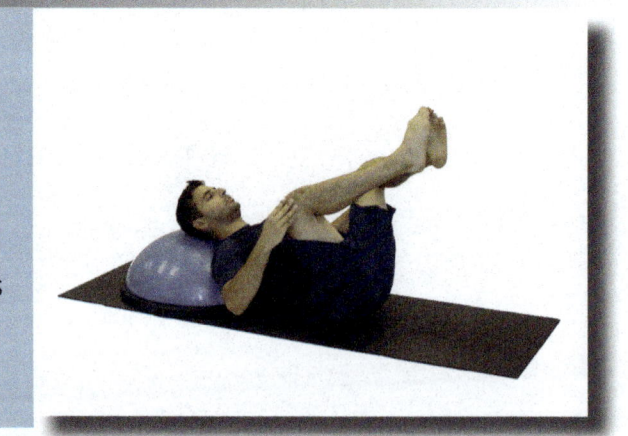

Exercise

Inhale	Lengthen the spine to prepare.
Exhale	Deepen the scoop in the lower belly (knees remain bent). Curl the head and shoulders off the dome.
Inhale	Simultaneously reach arms along the sides while legs extend up to ceiling. Hips rotate to parallel and feet flexed.
Exhale	Increase the abdominal scoop. Bend the knees, touching fingertips to the outside of the knees.
Inhale	Return to **Start Position**.
Reps	X5-10

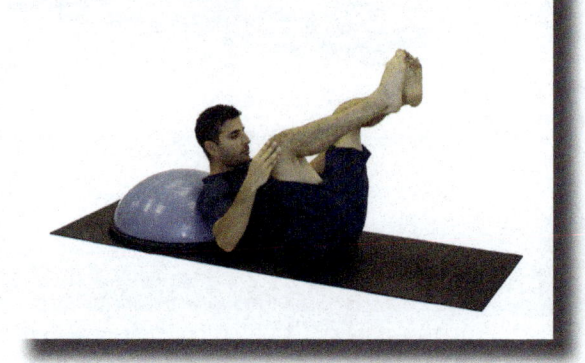

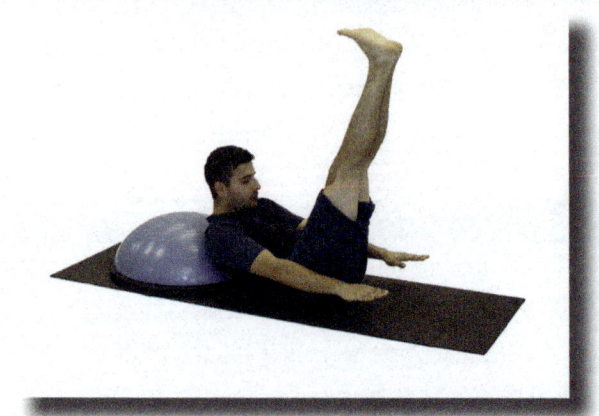

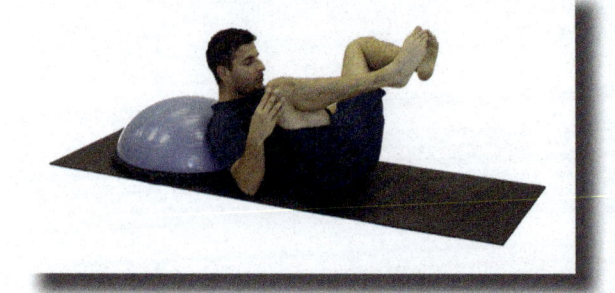

Modified

1. Head and shoulders on the mat, hips on dome. Bend and straighten the legs (Legs can be turned out or parallel when straight). Reps X5-10 (ASSIST)

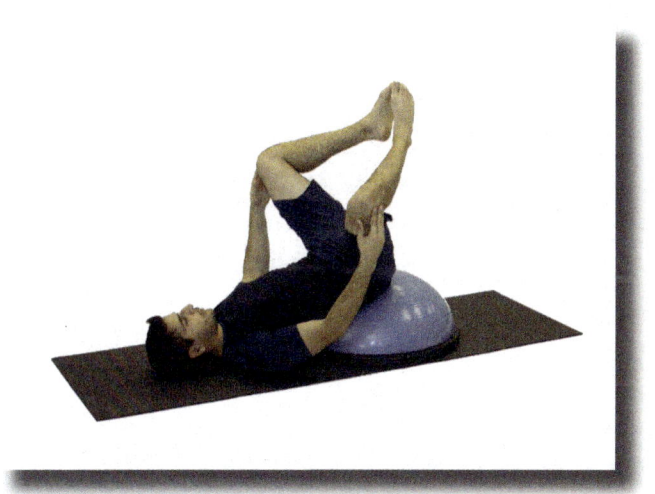

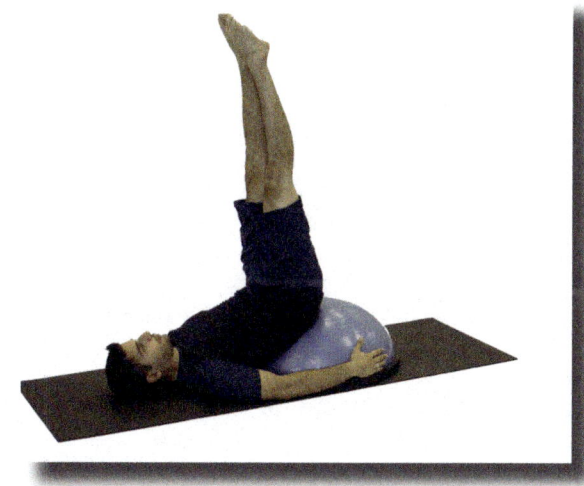

Muscular Intention

- Stabilizing the pelvis using abdominals, specifically the obliques and transverse abdominus during the leg extension.
- Co-ordinating the action of the hip flexors and hamstrings using adductors and abductors.
- Maintaining scapular depression using scapular stabilizers.

Tips

- ✔ Slide the shoulders down the back and keep the collar bones wide.
- ✔ Deepen the abdominal connection.
- ✔ Use the glutes to bend the legs and the hamstrings to extend the legs.

(39) FRONT LEG KICK

Start Position

1. Lying on R side over the top of the dome.
2. R forearm on the mat.
3. L hand on the dome.
4. R hip on the dome.
5. R knee bent.
6. L leg lifted and extended, with foot flexed.

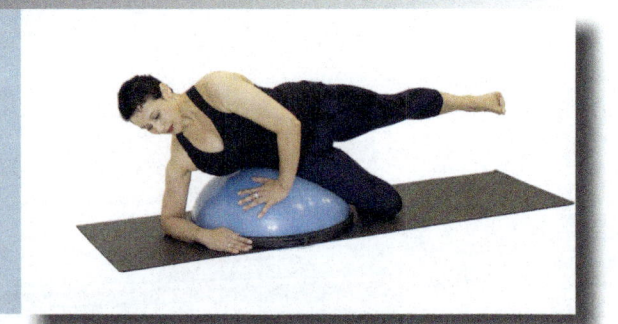

Exercise

Inhale   Flex L hip and bring the L leg forward. Pulse for two beats (flexed foot).

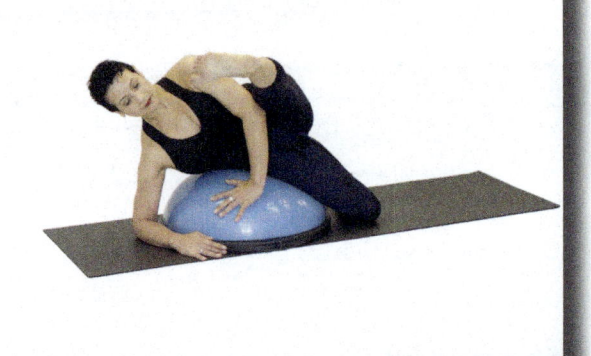

Exhale   Swing L leg back, extending L leg past the hips to the back. (pointed foot) Look back over the R shoulder.

Reps   X5-10

» Repeat on L side

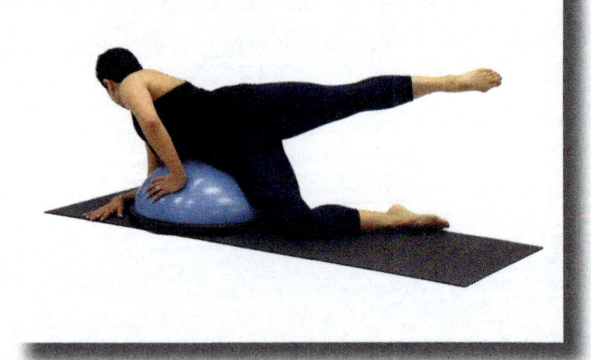

Modified

1. Pulse the L leg backwards. Foot flexed or pointed. Reps X5-10 L/R (CHALLENGE)

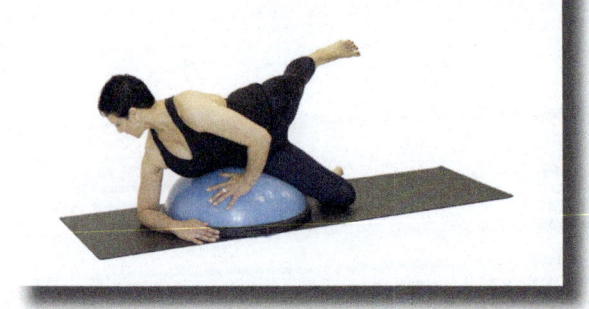

122 EXERCISES

Muscular Intention

- Stabilizing the hips using abdominals especially the internal abdominal obliques.
- Strengthening the flexors and extensors of the hips.
- Maintaining scapular depression using the scapular stabilizers.
- Lengthening the front of the thigh by connecting the glute and the hamstring.
- Strengthening the leg abductors of the working leg.

Tips

- ✔ Keep the hips stacked.
- ✔ Lengthen through the hamstring as you bring the top leg forward.
- ✔ Push the top hand into the dome and the forearm into the mat.
- ✔ Lift the chest as you look over the right shoulder.

FUNDAMENTALS

(40) SIDE BEND PREP

Start Position

1. Spine laterally flexed.
2. Sit on R hip away from the BOSU.
3. Knees are bent and feet flexed.
4. R foot is hooked behind a laterally rotated L foot on the mat.
5. L arm extended and touching the inside of the L knee.
6. R hand is on the dome.
7. R arm supports the torso.

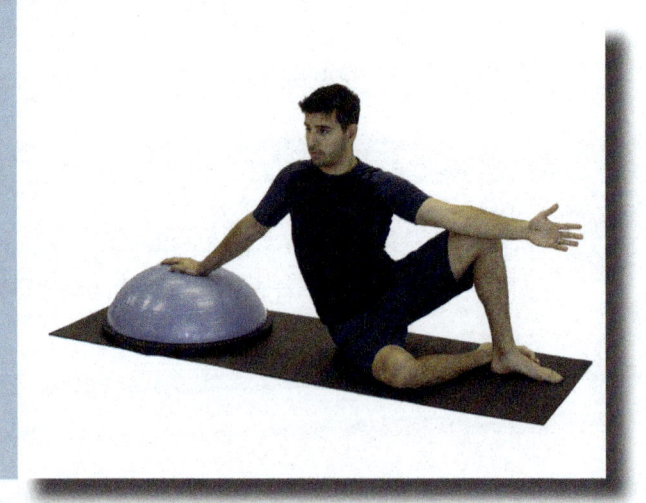

Exercise

Inhale   Press down into the R shin and lift hips off the floor. Reach the L arm to the ceiling while pressing down into the R hand. Keep both knees bent.

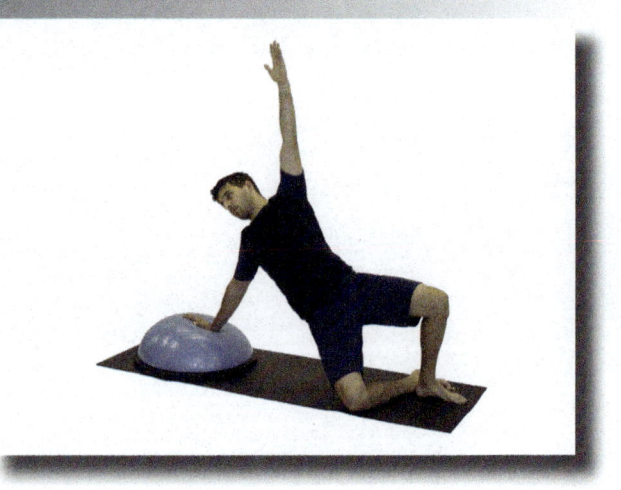

Exhale   Extend both legs and hook the R foot behind L foot while simultaneously reaching L arm overhead to open L ribs.

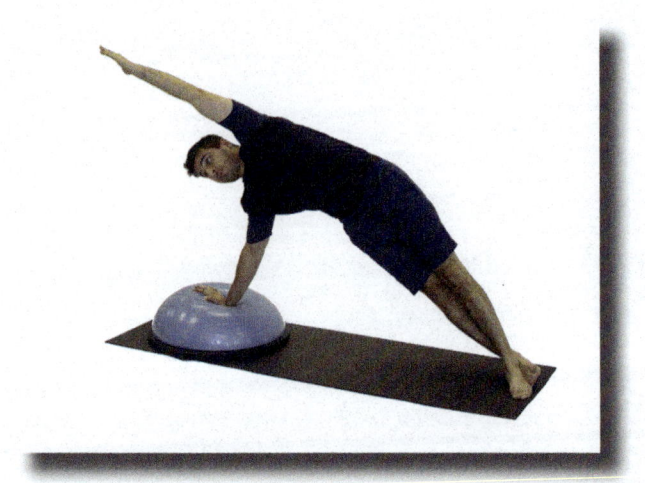

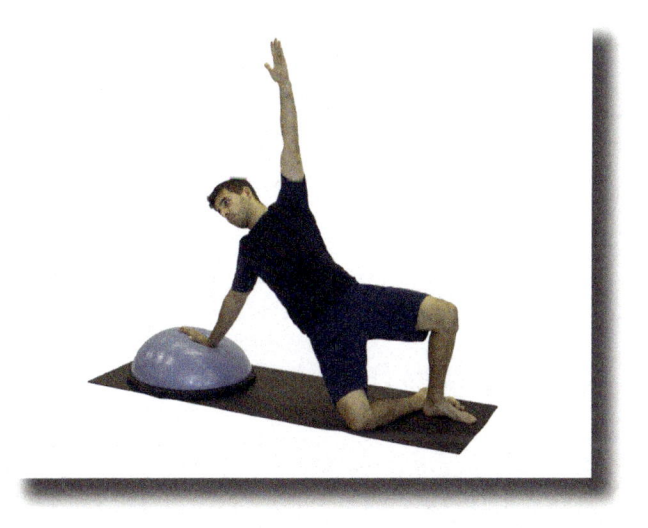

Inhale   Bring L arm to ceiling, bend both knees, hips still up.

Exhale   Return to **Start Position**.
Reps   X5 L/R

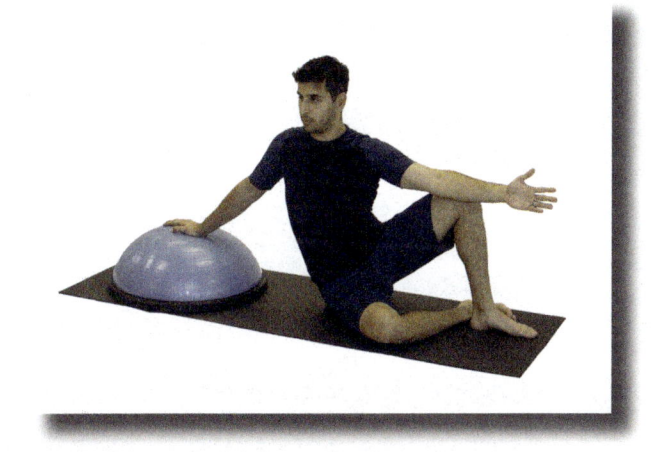

Modified

1. Keep bottom knee on the mat. Lift and lower the hips. Flex the R foot as you straighten the L leg. Reps X5 L/R (SIMPLIFY)

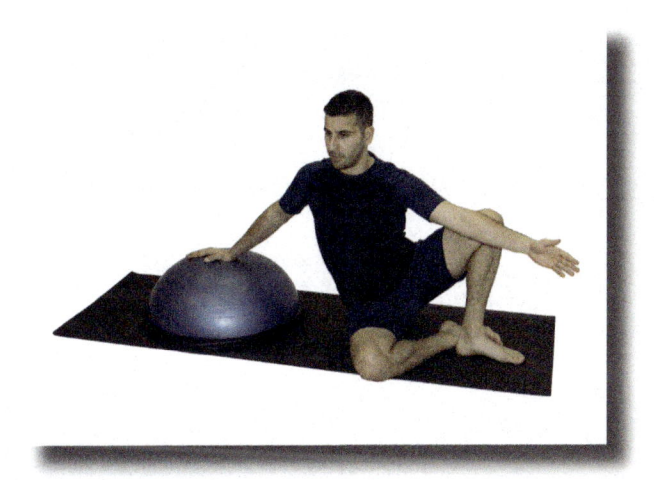

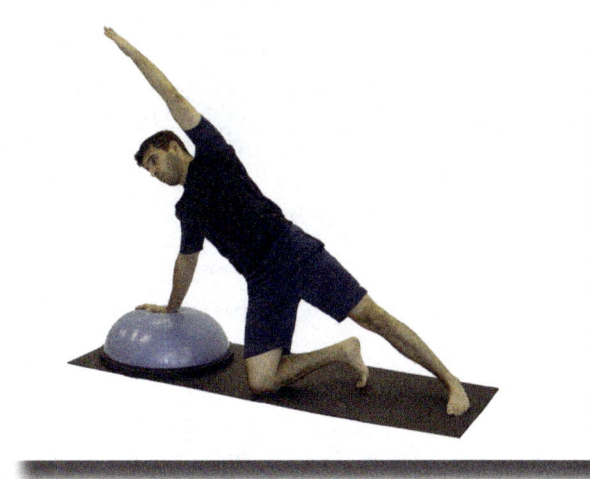

FUNDAMENTALS

2. On elbow into straight L leg, lift hips. Reach the L arm overhead. Keep the bottom knee on the mat. Reps X5-10 L/R (SIMPLIFY)

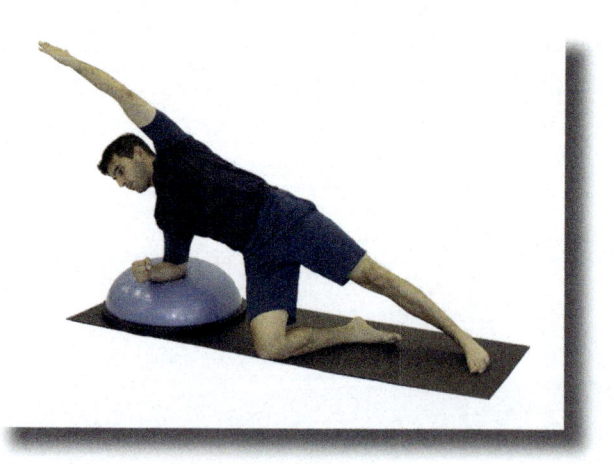

3. On elbow with hips up, kneel onto the R knee, straighten and hook the R foot behind the L foot. Return the R knee, keeping the hips up. Reps X5-10 L/R (CHALLENGE)

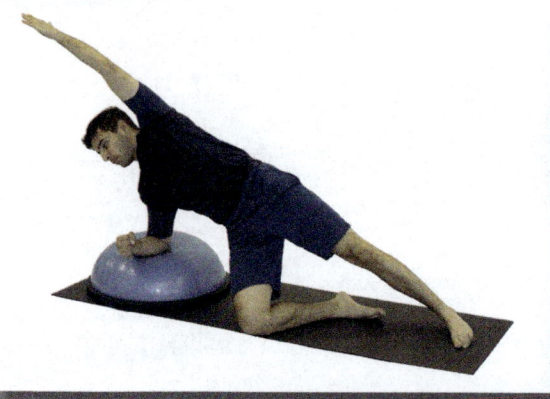

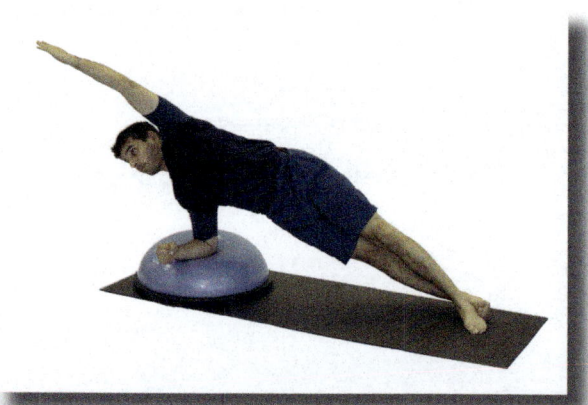

4. With hips down and knees stacked together, lift and lower the hips. Reps X5-10 L/R (SIMPLIFY)

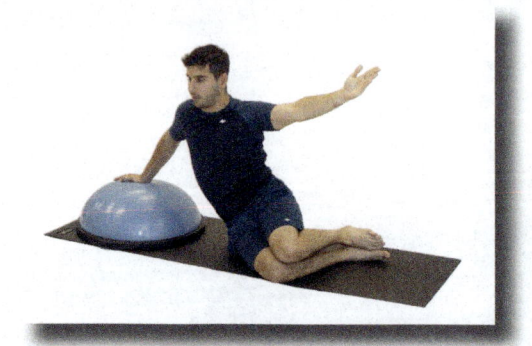

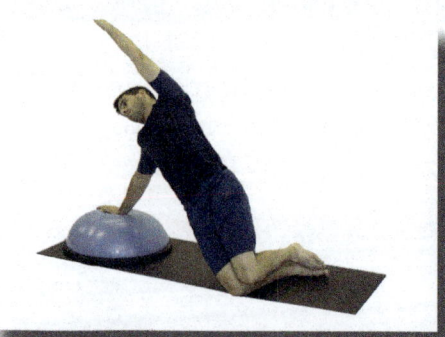

5. Place R foot on the dome, L hip, L knee and L hand on mat. R arm reaching overhead as you lift and lower the hips. Reps X5-10 L/R (SIMPLIFY)

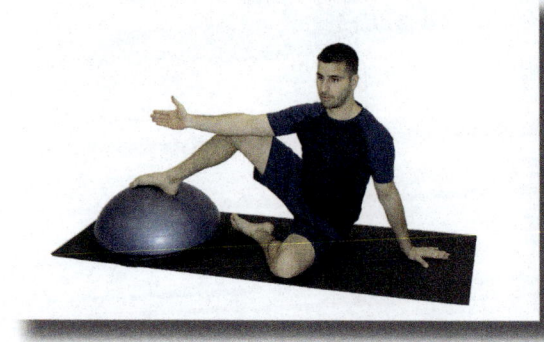

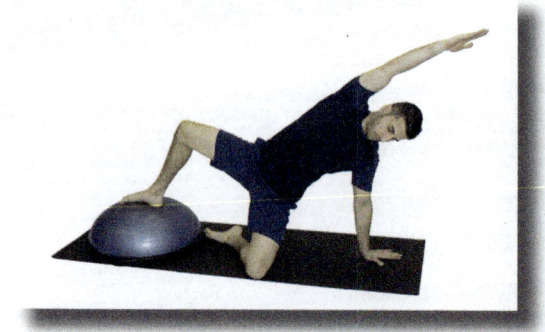

6. L elbow on the mat, R arm reaching in front of the R knee. R foot on the dome, L knee on the mat. Inhale to lift the hips and reach the R arm overhead. Exhale, extend and hook the L leg behind the R leg. Return to Start Position.
Reps X5-10 L/R (CHALLENGE)

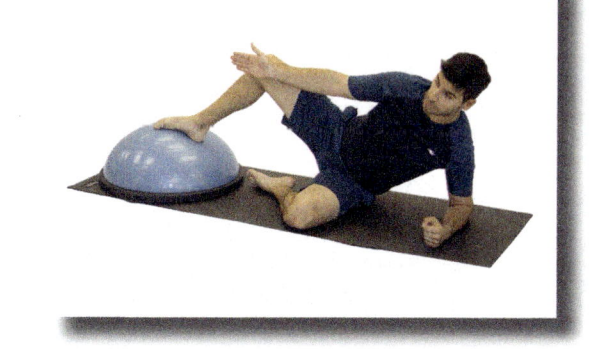

Hips elbow and knee on mat.

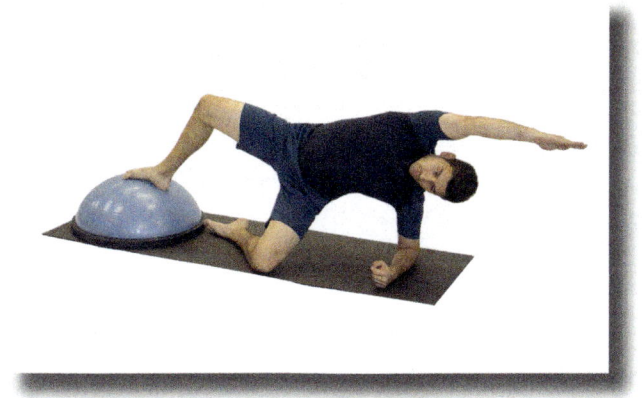

Lift hips and reach top arm overhead.

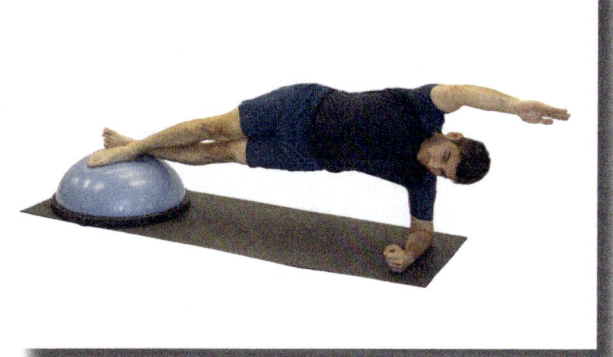

Hook L foot behind the R foot.

Muscular Intention

- Strengthening the hip flexors, quadriceps and adductors during the hip lift.
- Stabilizing the hips using the transverse abdominus and multifidi.
- Stabilizing the torso using the internal abdominal obliques to lift the hips.
- Maintaining scapular depression using the scapular stabilizers.

Tips

- ✔ Keep the hips stacked.
- ✔ Engage the lower abdominals.
- ✔ Look down the elbow/arm if you have any strain on the neck.
- ✔ Slide the shoulders down the back and keep the collar bones wide.
- ✔ Lean into the hand that is on the dome.

(41) SIDE ELBOW STRETCH WITH TWIST

Start Position

1. Spine laterally flexed.
2. Lie sideways with R elbow and forearm on the mat.
3. Place the R ribs and hip on the dome.
4. Bend the bottom knee with the L hip flexed.
5. L arm is extended overhead with palm facing down.
6. L leg is extended at hip height and foot pointed.

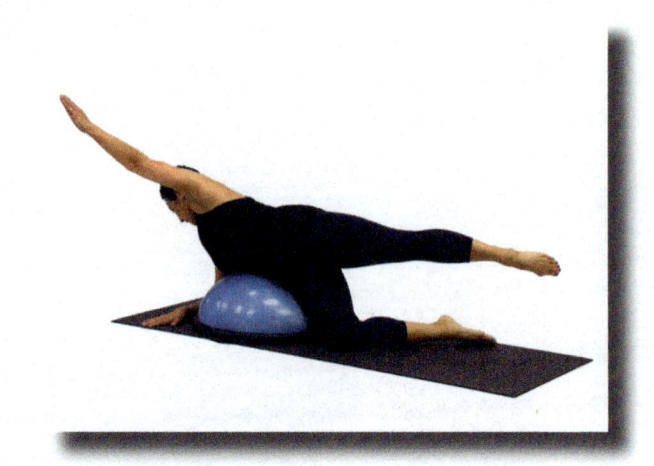

Exercise

Inhale   Extend and reach the L leg hovering at hip height. Reach the L arm overhead away from the L leg, looking down at the floor.

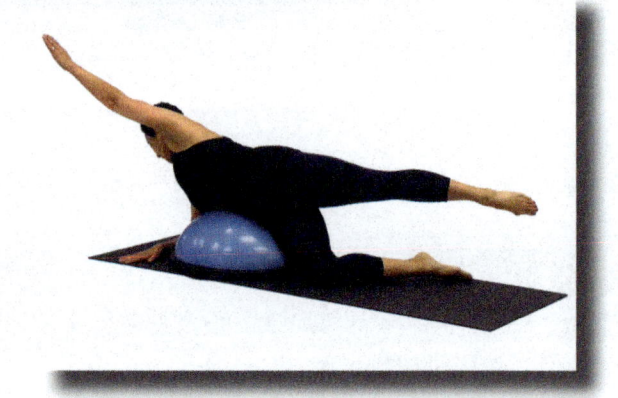

Exhale   Rotate the upper body even more and touch the L hand to R elbow, R hand to L elbow.

Inhale   Hold the position and breathe into the back for 4 breaths, while extending the L leg even further.

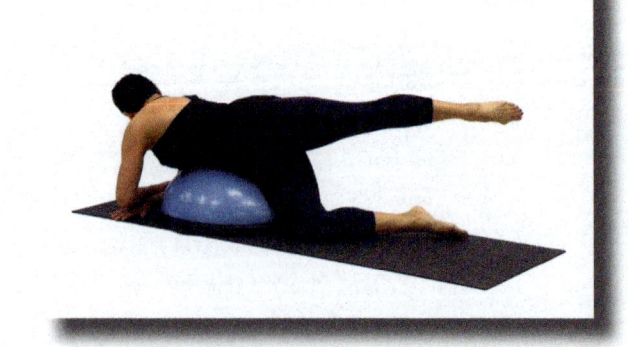

Exhale   Return sideways reaching the L arm overhead and extending the L leg. Repeat twist X5.

Inhale   Return to **Start Position**.

» Repeat on L side

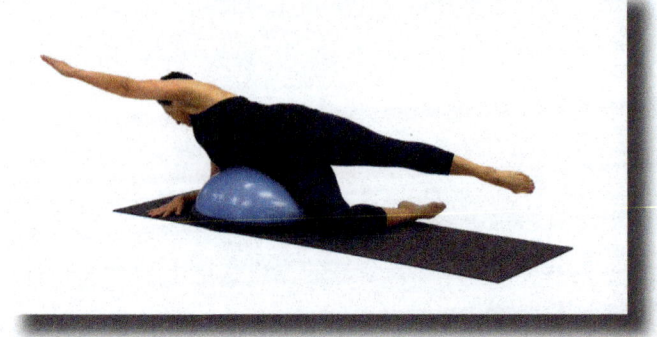

Modified

1. From bent knee and hand on the dome to extending the arm and the leg. Reps X10 (SIMPLIFY)

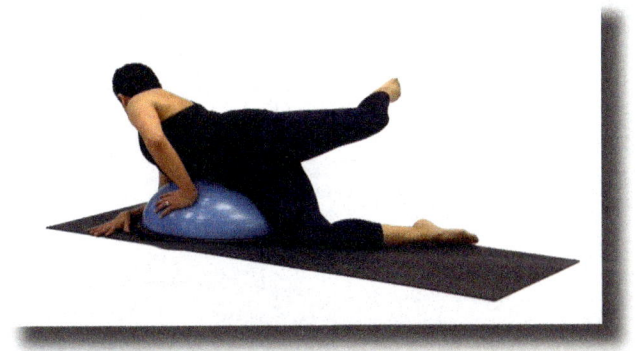

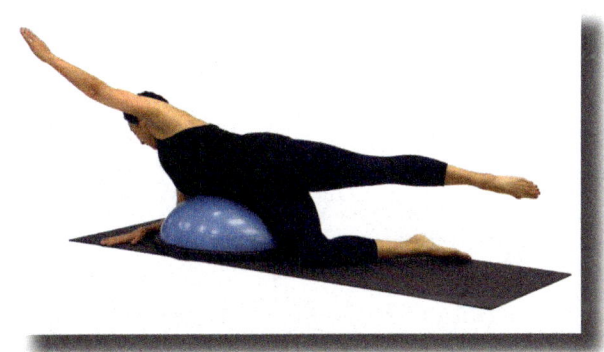

Muscular Intention

- Strengthening the spinal rotators by working the obliques and quadratus lumborum.
- Maintaining scapular depression using scapular stabilizers.
- Strengthening the hip extensors while reaching the leg backward.
- Strengthening the glutes and hamstrings during bending and straightening the leg.

Tips

- ✔ Slide the shoulders down the back and keep the collar bones wide.
- ✔ Press into the forearm as you lift the chest and look over your shoulder.
- ✔ Use the breath to deepen spinal rotation.
- ✔ Aim to keep both forearms on the mat.
- ✔ Extend the back leg away from the crown of the head.

(42) SIDE BEND WITH TWIST

Start Position

1. Spine laterally flexed.
2. Sit on R hip away from the BOSU.
3. Knees are bent and feet flexed.
4. R foot is hooked behind a laterally rotated L foot on the mat.
5. L arm extended and touching the inside of the L knee.
6. R hand is on the dome.
7. R arm supports the torso.

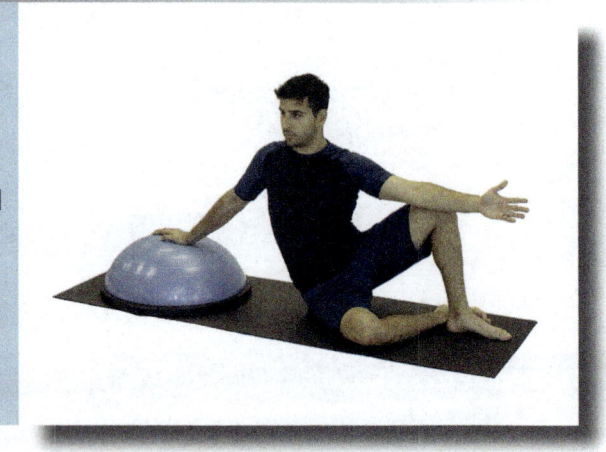

Exercise

Inhale   Lift the hips and reach L arm overhead while extending L leg. Keep R knee on the mat.

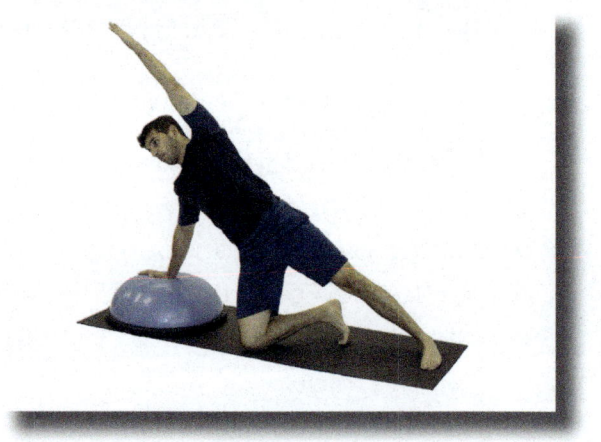

Exhale   Extend the R leg and hook the R foot behind the L foot. Lift the hips to the ceiling and bring the L hand underneath the torso. Look down at the floor.

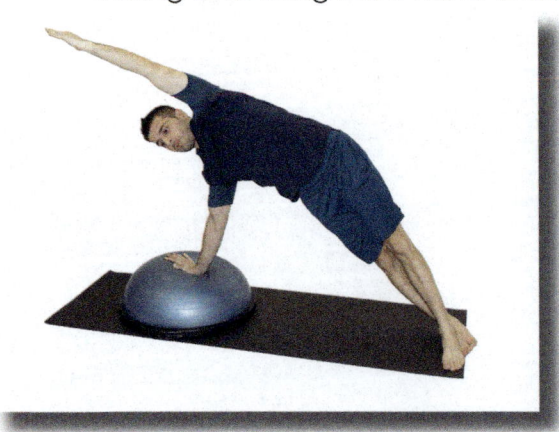

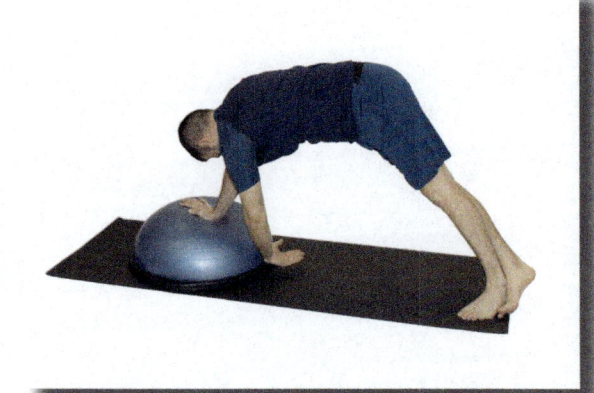

Inhale   Return the L arm overhead. Spine is laterally flexed, facing forward.

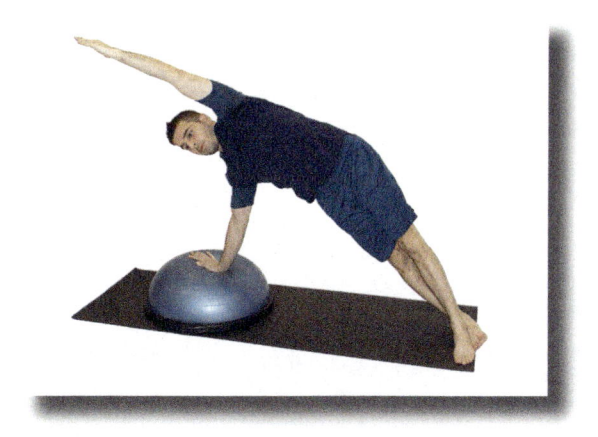

Exhale   Return to **Start Position**.
Reps   X5 L/R

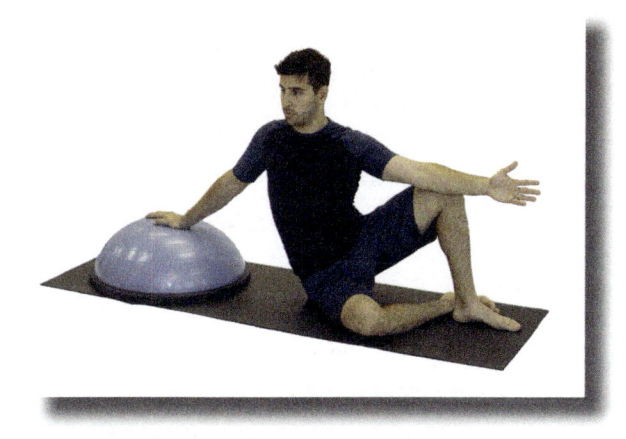

Modified

1. Do side bend only, with arm overhead and two straight legs. Return to **Start Position** and repeat. Reps X5 (SIMPLIFY)

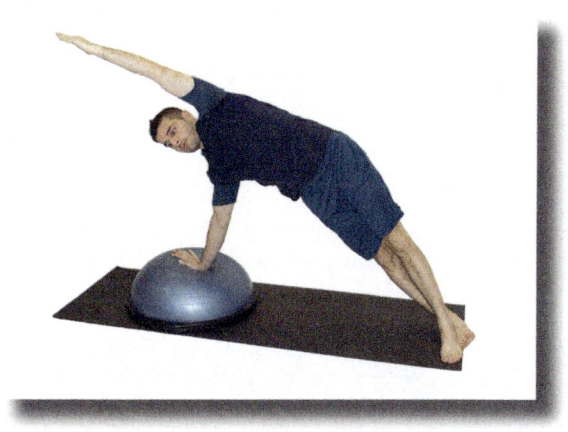

2. Start kneeling on R knee with elbow on the dome, L leg extended, L arm overhead. Extend the R leg and hook the R foot behind the L foot. Hips up. Return R knee to mat. Reps X5 then return to **Start Position.** (CHALLENGE)

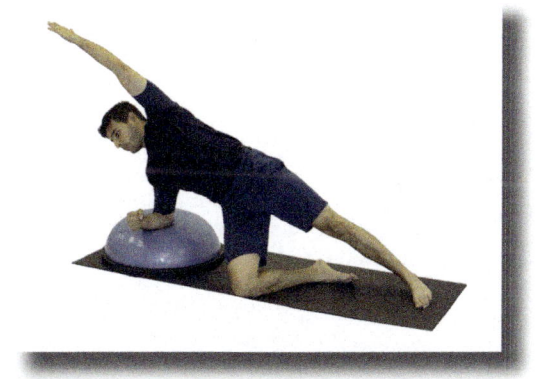

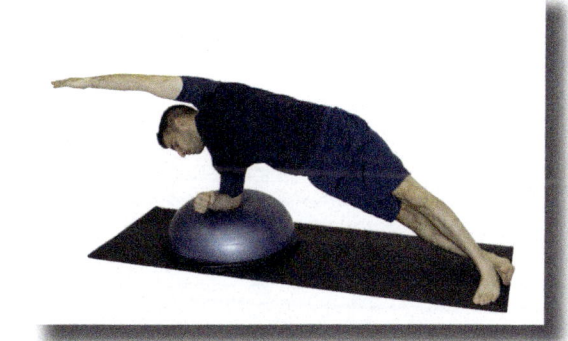

FUNDAMENTALS   131

3. Flat side up. R hand on flat side. Keep the knees bent. Lift and lower the hips only
Reps X5 (SIMPLIFY)

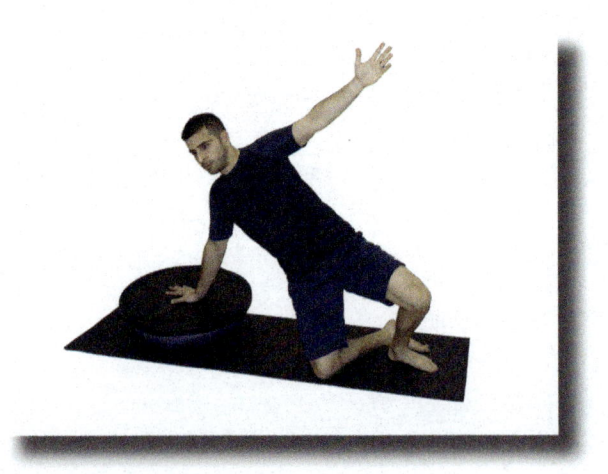

Muscular Intention

- Strengthening the spinal rotators by working the obliques and quadratus lumborum.
- Maintaining scapular depression using scapular stabilizers.
- Strengthening the leg abductors and adductors when the legs come together.

Tips

- ✔ Slide the shoulders down the back and keep the collar bones wide.
- ✔ Press down into the hand as you lift the hips.
- ✔ Use the breath to deepen spinal rotation and lateral flexion.
- ✔ Squeeze the inner thighs together as you hook the bottom foot behind the top foot.
- ✔ Lift the bottom hip as you bring the top arm underneath the ribs.
- ✔ During the side bend, separate the top arm away from the top leg.

(43) PILATES PUSH-UP PREP 2

Start Position

1. Spine neutral.
2. Standing about one foot away from the BOSU.
3. Hands along the sides.
4. Feet together.

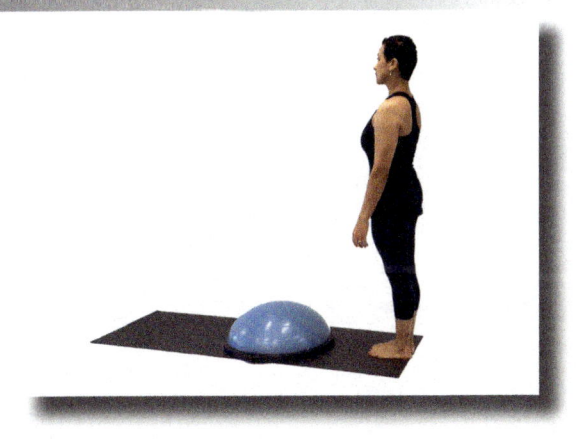

Exercise

Inhale   Lengthen the spine.

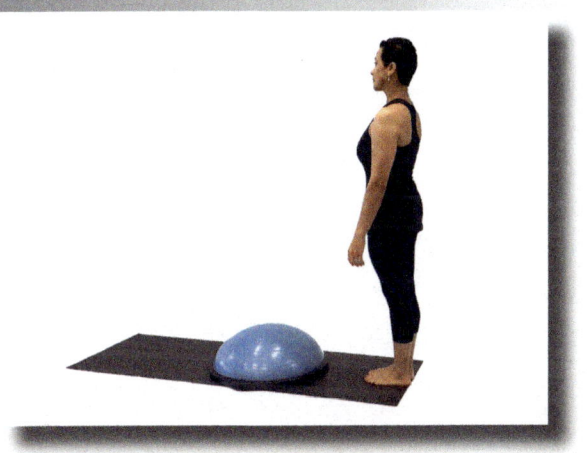

Exhale   Curl the upper body forward starting from the top of the head.

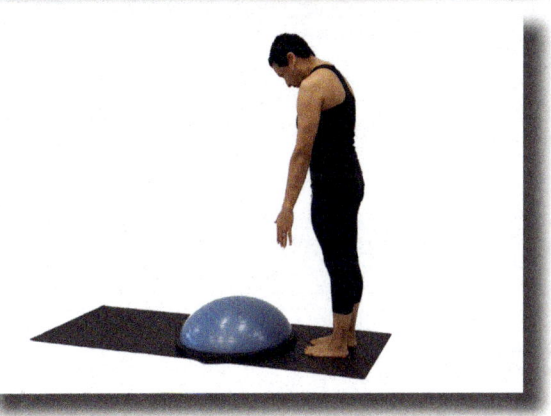

Inhale   Place both hands on the dome and hold. Breathe into the lower back.

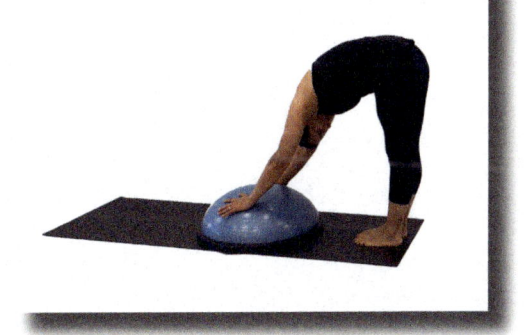

FUNDAMENTALS   133

Exhale   Using the abdominals lift and lower the heels X5.

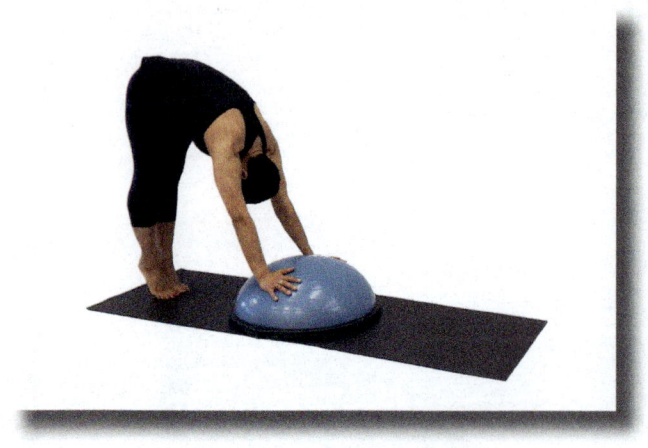

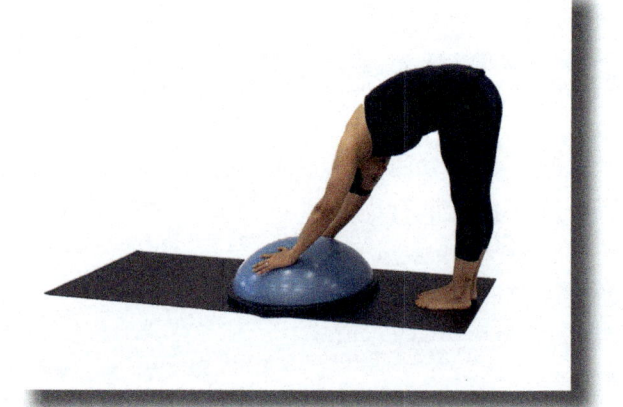

Then...

Inhale   Lift both heels and lower the knees to the dome, deepening the abdominal curl.

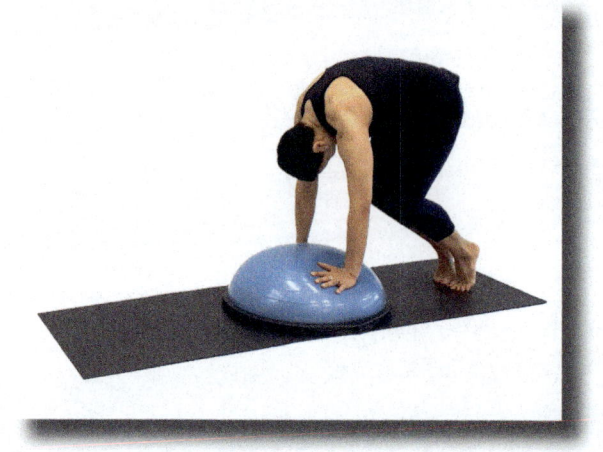

Exhale   Continue to lower knees to hands on the dome.

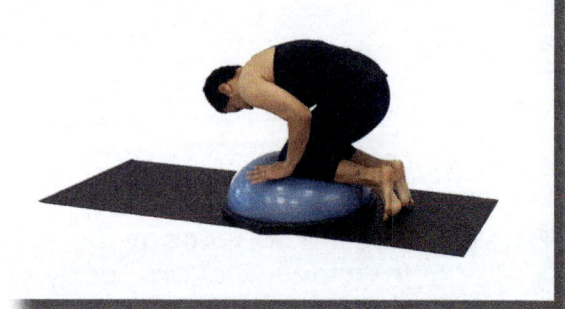

Inhale   Start to walk the hands forward along the mat away from BOSU, until torso is in a straight line in plank position.

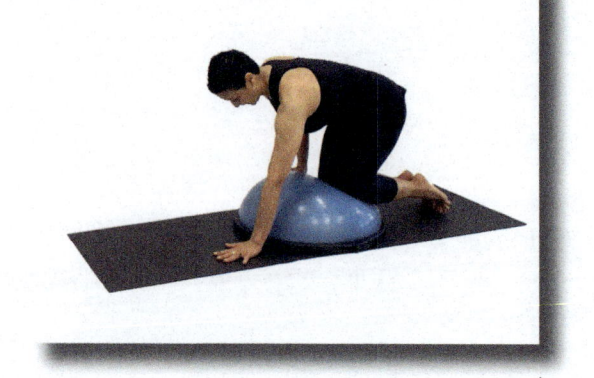

Walk out with one hand at a time.

134   **EXERCISES**

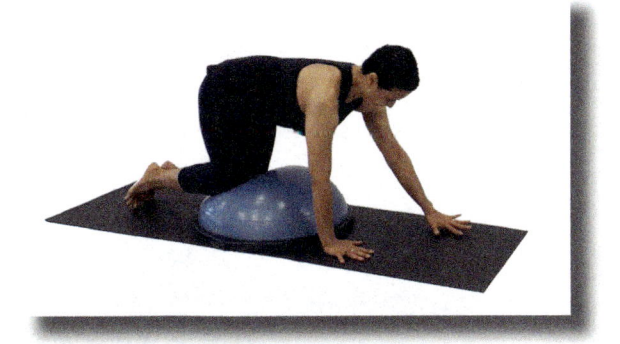

Start to lean the hips forward.

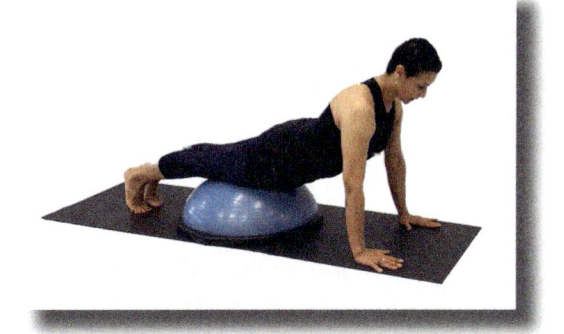

Into plank with hips down.

Exhale   Lift the head and chest to ceiling.

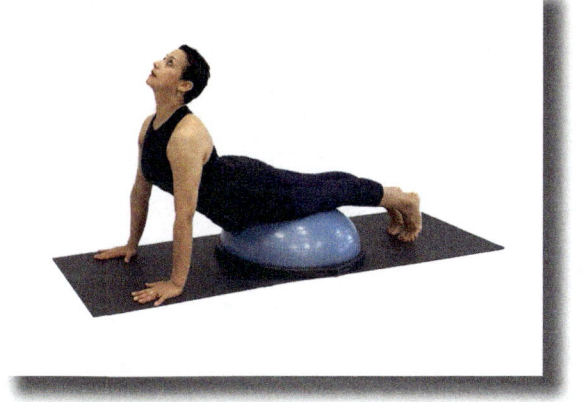

Inhale   Return head in line with spine and lift the hips into plank, knees off the dome.

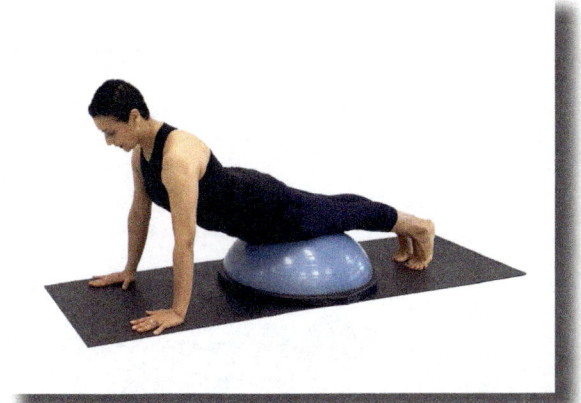

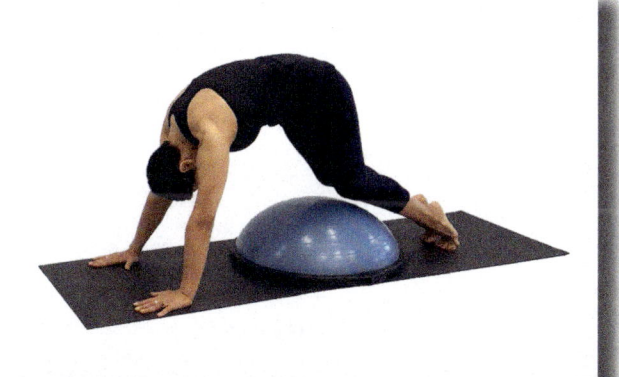

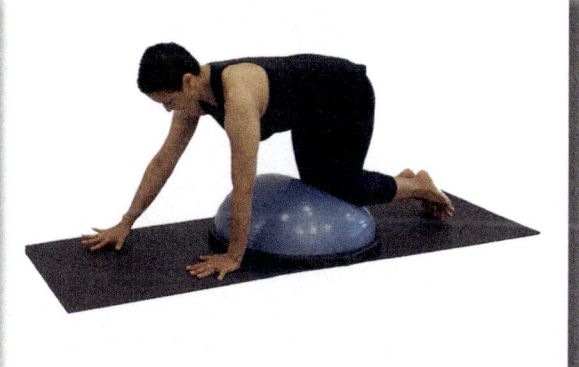

Exhale   Place the knees back onto the dome and walk hands back toward the knees.

FUNDAMENTALS 135

Inhale   Keep the toes tucked under and place both hands onto the dome.

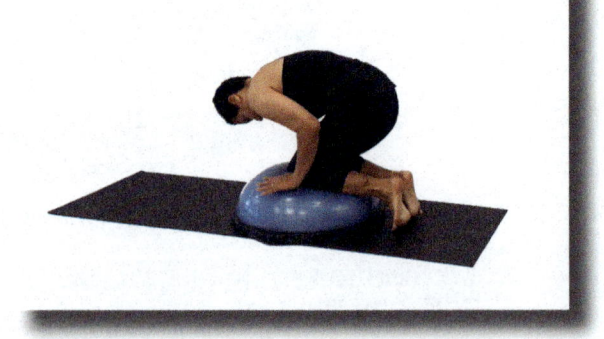

Exhale   Push into the dome with hands and extend the legs.
Inhale   Roll up through the spine to **Start Position.**
Reps   X5-10

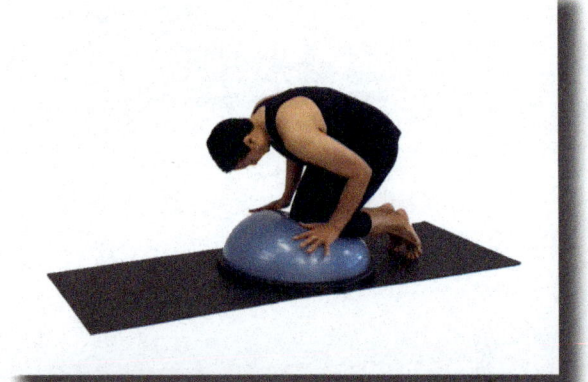

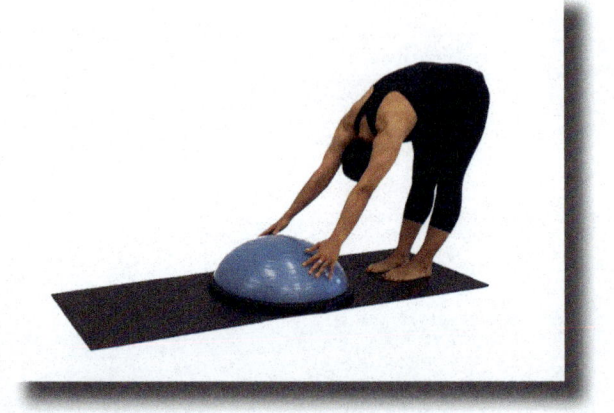

Modified

1. Push-up position. Lift knees and lower the knees, hands on the mat. Reps X10 (ASSIST)

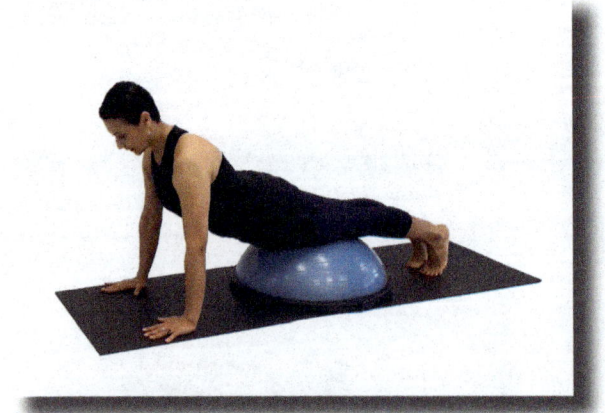

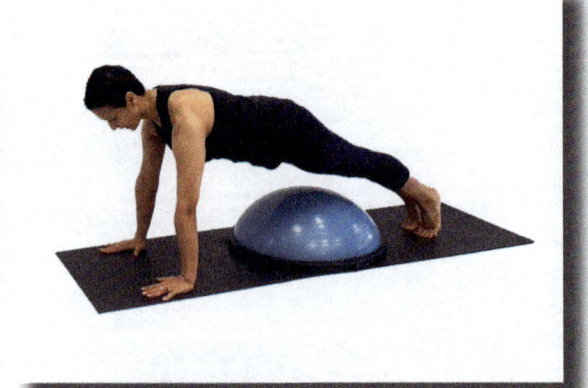

136 EXERCISES

2. Hands on the dome, lower knees toward the dome, then straighten both legs. Reps X5. (SIMPLIFY)

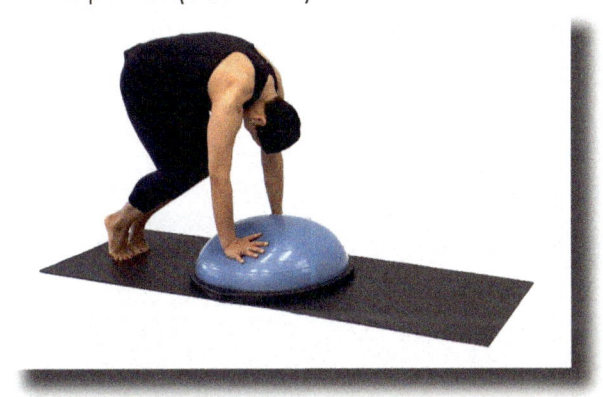

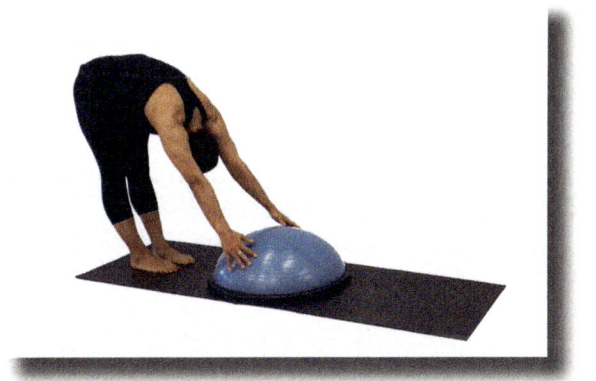

3. Lift the hips into a pike (downward dog position), then into plank position with hips above the BOSU. Reps X5 (CHALLENGE)

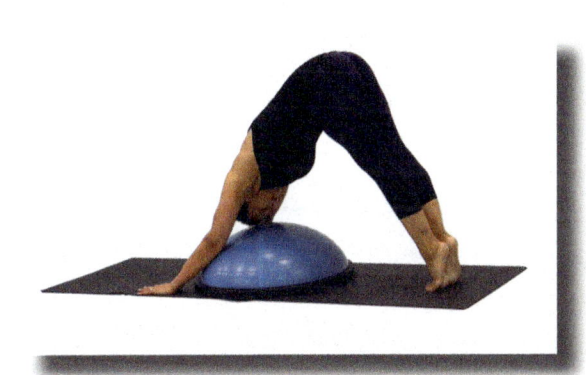

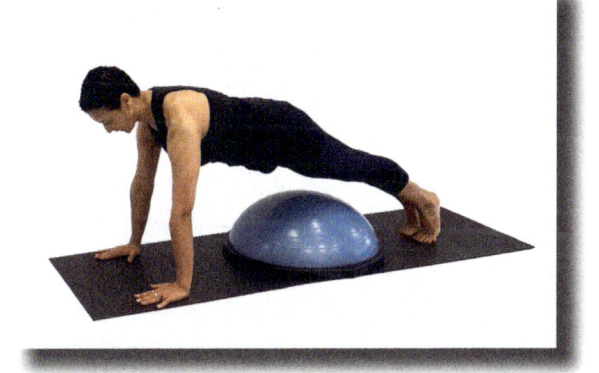

4. Start in plank. Keep knees on the dome and extend the spine in the Cobra looking up. Return to plank. Reps X5 (SIMPLIFY)

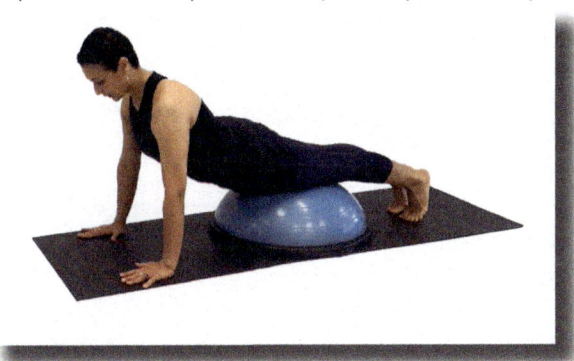

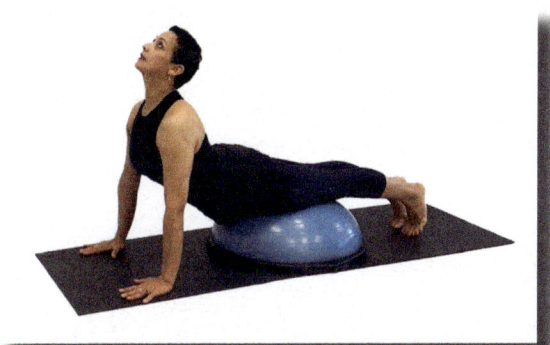

FUNDAMENTALS

Muscular Intention

- Connecting the shoulder blades by using the latissimus dorsi and serratus posterior and anterior.
- Stabilizing the torso using the deep abdominals and paraspinals.
- Stretching the paraspinals by using the abdominals in the roll down.

Tips

- ✔ Push hands into the dome (or into the floor).
- ✔ Increase the abdominal connection during the heel lifts.
- ✔ Slide the shoulders down the back and keep the collar bones wide (during the plank and cobra).
- ✔ Push the dome away from the chest with hands and lift the hips to ceiling. (Pike)
- ✔ Knit the ribs toward the hips during the plank.

(44) SEAL

Start Position

1. Spine imprinted.
2. Sit in front of the BOSU on the mat, lower back against the dome.
3. Knees bent and wider than shoulder width.
4. Soles of feet together.
5. Hands hold under ankles, from the inside of thighs.
6. Press elbows against the knees and knees against the elbows.

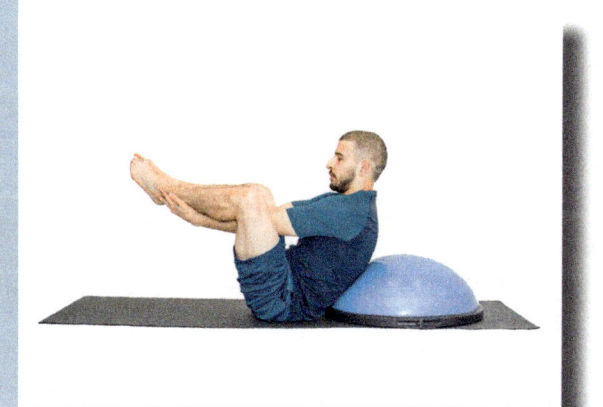

Exercise

Inhale	Increase the C shape.
Exhale	Hold position and come away from the dome.

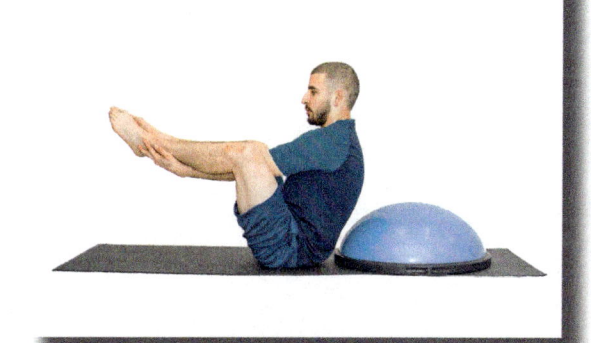

Inhale	Return to **Start Position** – lower back against the dome.
Reps	X10

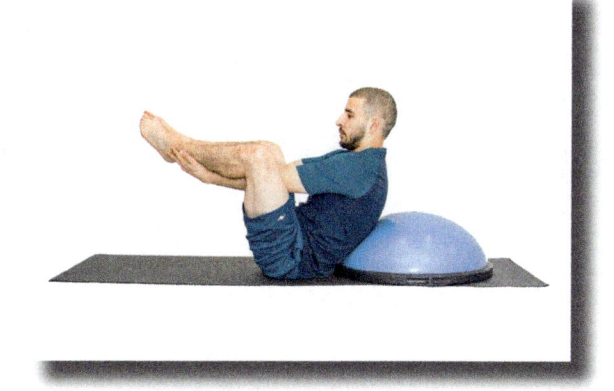

Modified

1. Hands hold ankles or calves from the outside of both legs. Reps X10 (SIMPLIFY)

FUNDAMENTALS 139

2. Feet clap 3 times for balance and control. Sit further away from the dome. Reps X10 (CHALLENGE)

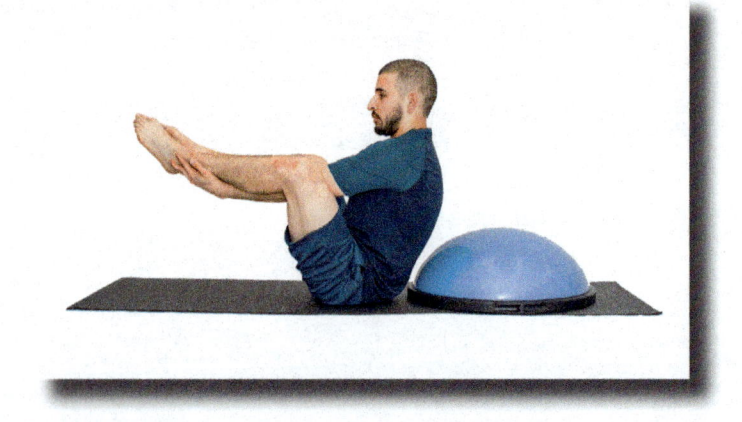

Muscular Intention
- Stabilizing the pelvis against the hip flexors using the abdominals.
- Maintaining scapular depression using scapular stabilizers.
- Strengthening and stabilizing the abductors and adductors of the arms and legs.

Tips
- ✔ Slide the shoulders down the back and keep the collar bones wide.
- ✔ Deepen the abdominal connection using the breath during the balance.
- ✔ Keep the knees a comfortable distance from the chest.
- ✔ Press the arms against the legs and legs against the arms.

(45) MERMAID

Start Position

1. Sit sideways against the BOSU on R hip.
2. R hand resting on the dome.
3. L arm reaching out to the side at shoulder height, palm up.
4. Knees bent, both feet to the L side.

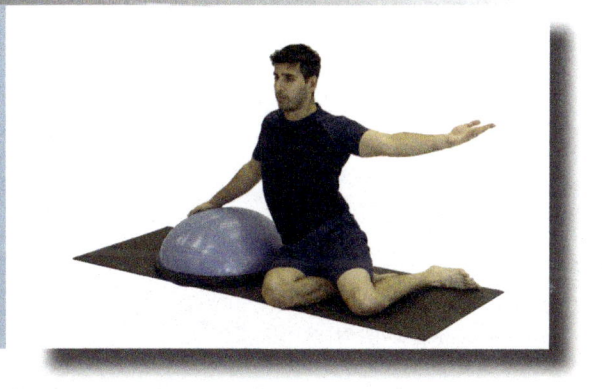

Exercise

Inhale — Lift L arm overhead and reach up toward the ceiling.

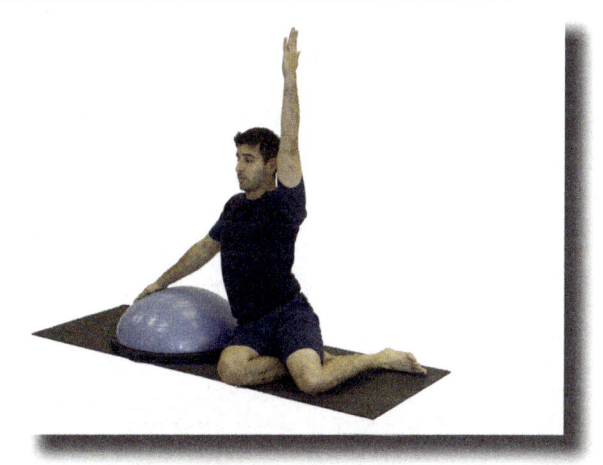

Exhale — Side bend over the dome, R hand on the mat – reaching L arm overhead.

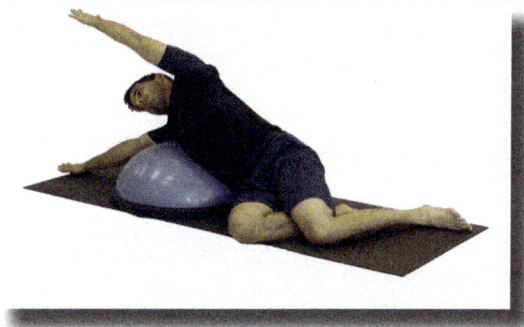

Inhale — Use R arm to assist the torso and lifting the L arm to the ceiling and return to sitting position.

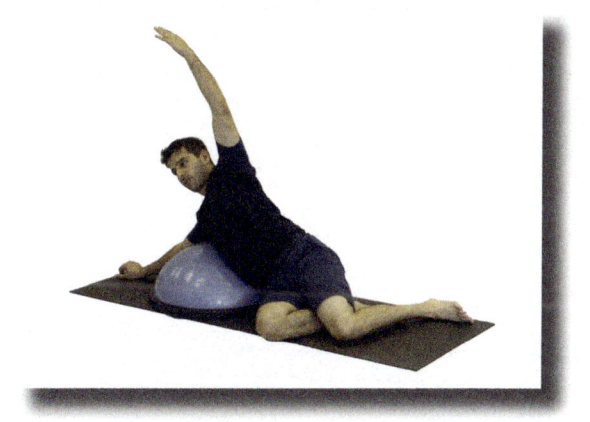

FUNDAMENTALS 141

Exhale   Return R hand to the dome to **Start Position**.

Reps   X5 L/R

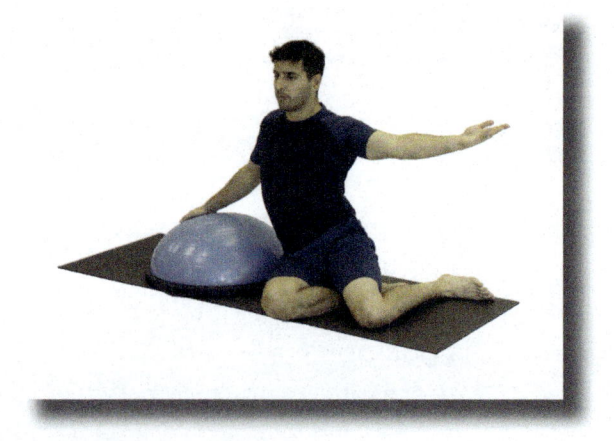

Modified

1. Side stretch over the dome with R hand supporting the head. Lean back and reach the L arm diagonally overhead. Hold the position for 5 breaths.
   Reps L/R (CHALLENGE)

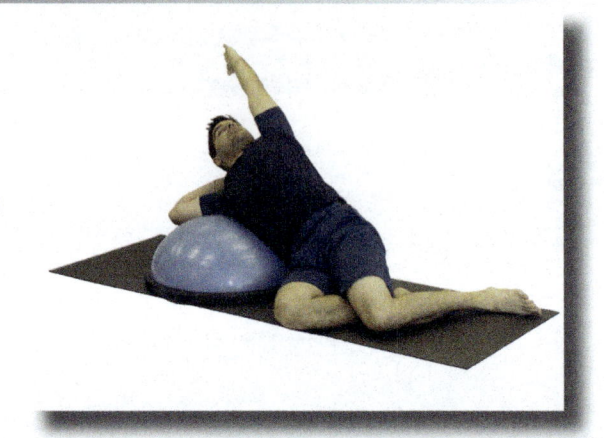

Muscular Intention

- Stretching the quadratus lumborum and latissimus dorsi.
- Maintaining scapular depression using scapular stabilizers.
- Stretching and lengthening the deep intercostal muscles.

Tips

✔ Keep the hips stacked.
✔ Engage the lower abdominals during the side bend.
✔ Separate the top hip from the bottom rib.
✔ Deepen the abdominal connection using the breath.

REFERENCE CHART

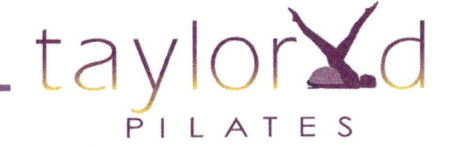

	Exercise	BOSU Placement	Reps
Warm Up:			
1.	Spinal Mobilization	Dome	X5
2.	Hip Release	Dome	X5
3.	Arch and Curl Spine	Dome	X5
4.	Circle Upper Body	Dome	X5 L/R
5.	Tip Upper Body Side to Side	Dome	X5 L/R
6.	Scapulae Isolations	Dome	X5-10
7.	Arms Circles	Dome	X5-10
The Workout			
8.	Abdominals	Dome	X5-10
9.	Breast Stroke Prep	Dome	X5-10
10.	Child's Pose	Dome	X5 Breaths
11.	Hundred	Dome/Flat	X10 Cycles
12.	Half Roll Back	Dome	X5
13.	Roll Up Prep	Dome	X5-10
14.	Single Leg Circle	Dome	X5 CW/CCW R/L
15.	Sitting Spine Twist	Dome/Flat	X5 L/R
16.	Side Lying Lateral Obliques	Dome	X10 R/L
17.	Single Leg Stretch Prep	Dome	X10 Sets
18.	Double Leg Stretch Prep	Dome/Flat	X10
19.	Scissors Prep	Dome	X10 Sets
20.	Shoulder Bridge Prep	Dome/Flat	X5-10
21.	Roll Over Prep	Dome	X5-10
22.	Double Leg Extension Prep	Dome	X5-10
23.	Single Leg Kick	Dome	X5 L/R
24.	Saw	Dome/Flat	X5 L/R
25.	Neck Pull Prep	Dome	X5
26.	Obliques Roll Back	Dome	X10 L/R
27.	Teaser Prep	Dome/Flat	X5-10 Sets
28.	Side Lying Clam Series	Dome	X5-10 L/R
29.	Side Leg Lift Series	Dome	X10 L/R
30.	Cat Stretch	Dome/Flat	X5
31.	Sitting Spine Stretch Forward	Dome/Flat	X5
32.	Swan Dive Prep	Dome	X10
33.	Swimming Prep	Dome/Flat	X10 L/R
34.	Leg Pull Front Prep	Dome/Flat	X10
35.	Reverse Plank Prep (Leg Pull)	Dome/Flat	X5
36.	Pilates Push-Up Prep 1	Dome/Flat	X5
37.	Elbow Plank Prep	Dome	X5-10
38.	Slow Double Leg Stretch Prep	Dome	X5-10
39.	Front Leg Kick	Dome	X5-10 R/L
40.	Side Bend Prep	Dome	X5 L/R
41.	Side Elbow Stretch with Twist	Dome	X5 L/R
42.	Side Bend with Twist	Dome/Flat	X5 L/R
43.	Pilates Push-Up Prep 2	Dome	X5-10
44.	Seal	Dome	X5
45.	Mermaid	Dome	X5 L/R

FUNDAMENTALS

taylor d
PILATES
www.taylor-dpilates.com

GLOSSARY

BODY PARTS

Abdominals

A large group of muscles in the front of the abdomen that assists in the regular breathing movement and supports the muscles of the spine while lifting and keeping abdominal organs such as the intestines in place.

Internal Abdominal Obliques
External Abdominal Obliques
Rectus Abdominus
Transverse Abdominus

- Internal Obliques
- External Obliques
- Rectus Abdominus
- Transverse Abdominus

Abductors of the Legs

Muscles of the outer thigh that assist in reaching the legs away from the midline. Both abductors and adductors assist in stabilizing the pelvis during walking.

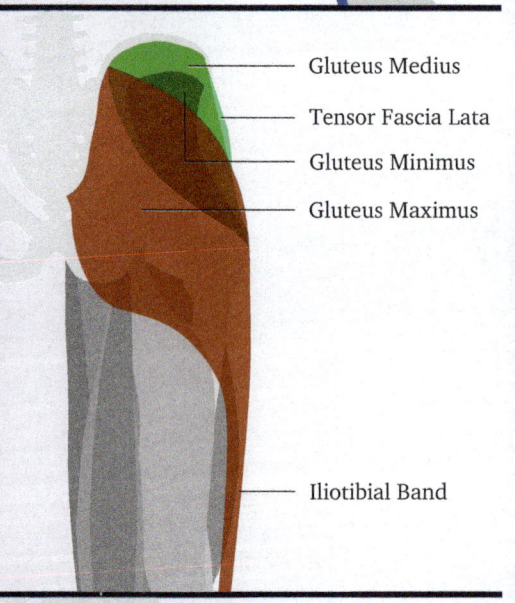

- Gluteus Medius
- Tensor Fascia Lata
- Gluteus Minimus
- Gluteus Maximus
- Iliotibial Band

Adductors of the Legs

Muscles of the inner thigh that assist in bringing the legs together toward the mid line. Both abductors and adductors assist in stabilizing the pelvis during walking.

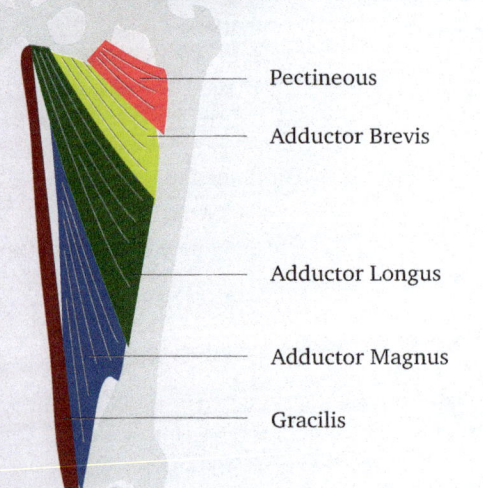

- Pectineous
- Adductor Brevis
- Adductor Longus
- Adductor Magnus
- Gracilis

144 EXTRAS

Back Extensors

These muscles are attached to the back of the spine. The back extensors keep the back erect in proper posture. The back muscles will include:

Latissimus Dorsi
Serratus Posterior
Rhomboids
Paraspinals

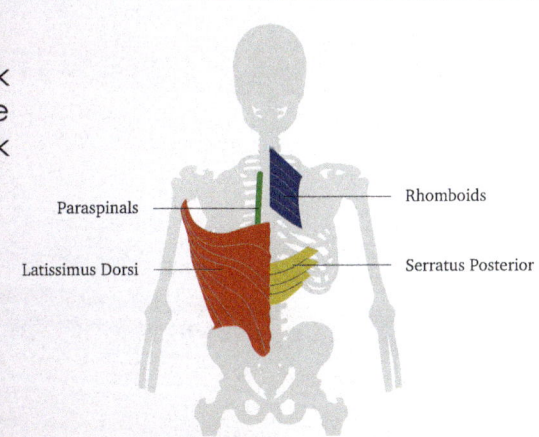

Paraspinals, Rhomboids, Latissimus Dorsi, Serratus Posterior

Cervical Spine

The neck bones, consisting of seven vertebrae, and sits between the cranium (skull bone) and the thoracic spine.

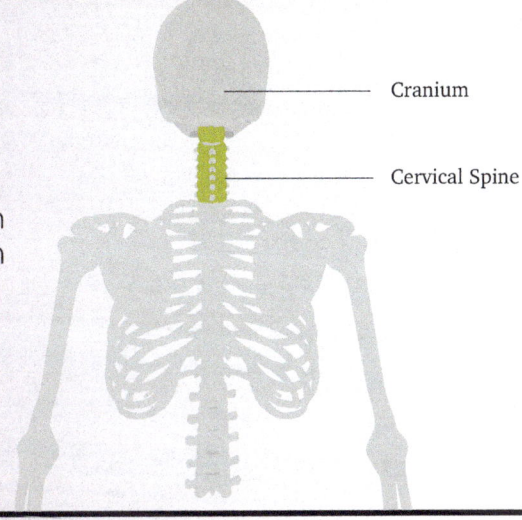

Cranium, Cervical Spine

Collarbones

The Collar Bone is also referred to as the Clavicle. It is a long, thin bone, "S" shaped, that connects the arm to the trunk. It is located directly above the first rib and acts as a strut to keep the scapula in place so that the arm can hang freely.

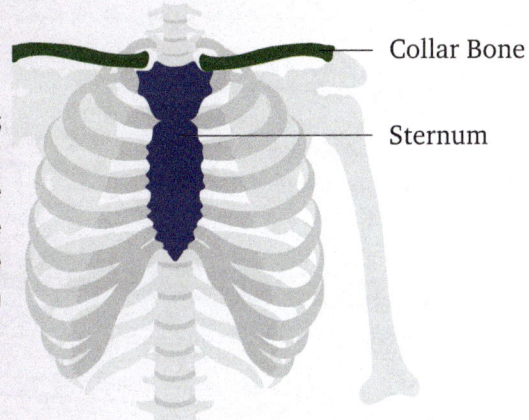

Collar Bone, Sternum

FUNDAMENTALS

External Abdominal Obliques

The muscles at the side of the abdominals that twist or rotate the spine. External Abdominal Obliques help to stabilize the hips. Working together, the larger External Abdominal Obliques covers the Internal Abdominal Obliques

— External Obliques

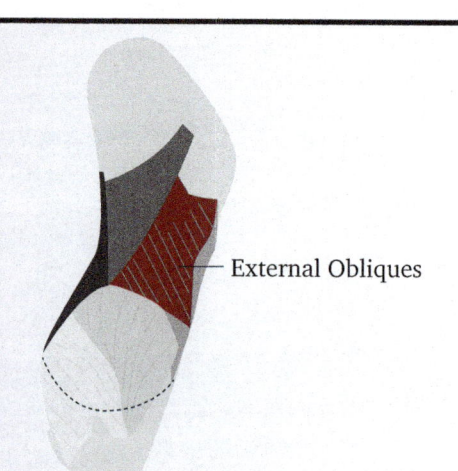

Foot Extensors

The muscles in the back of the lower legs and feet, that help to point the feet.

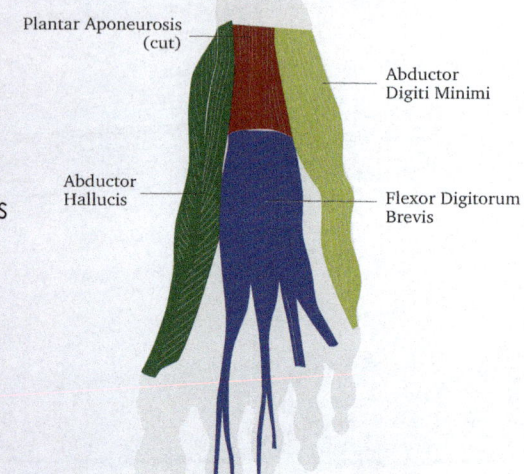

Plantar Aponeurosis (cut)
Abductor Digiti Minimi
Abductor Hallucis
Flexor Digitorum Brevis

Foot Flexors

The muscles in the back of the lower legs and feet, that help to flex the feet.

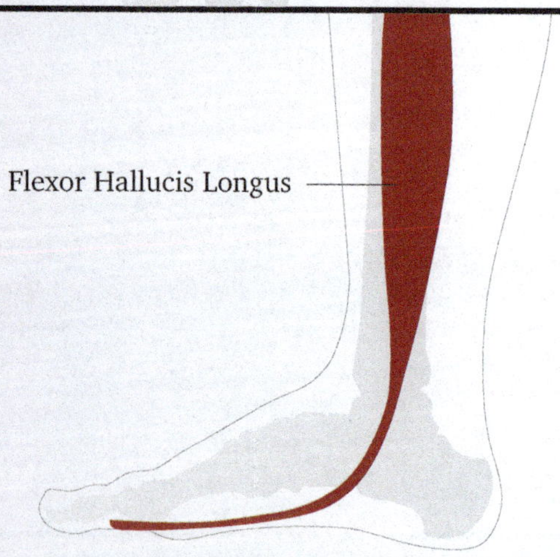

Flexor Hallucis Longus

146 **EXTRAS**

Gluteals (Glutes)	The muscle group of the buttocks, that contribute to hip movement and pelvic/back stability. Consists of 3 muscles.	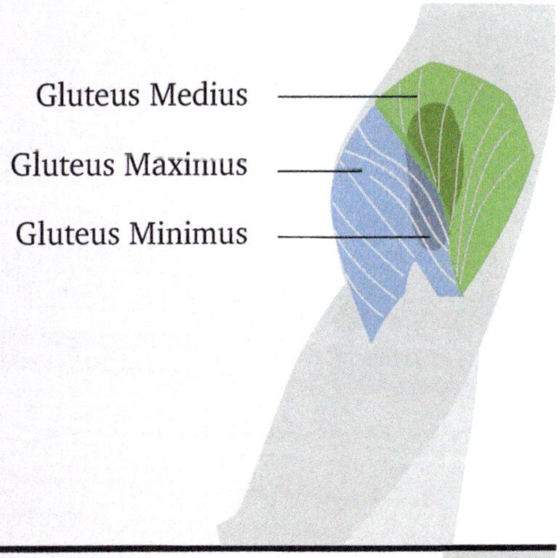 Gluteus Medius Gluteus Maximus Gluteus Minimus
Hamstrings	A group of three muscles at the back of the thigh, or upper leg, extending from the sitting bone connecting to the head of the tibia (shin bone) and fibula (calf bone). Hamstrings bend the knee and assist in backwards leg motion and includes walking, squatting and tilting the pelvis.	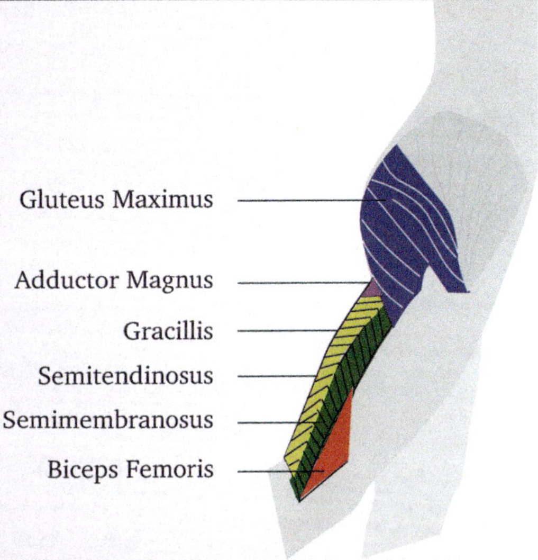 Gluteus Maximus Adductor Magnus Gracillis Semitendinosus Semimembranosus Biceps Femoris
Hips	A projection of the pelvis and upper thigh bone.0 (femur) on each side of the body.	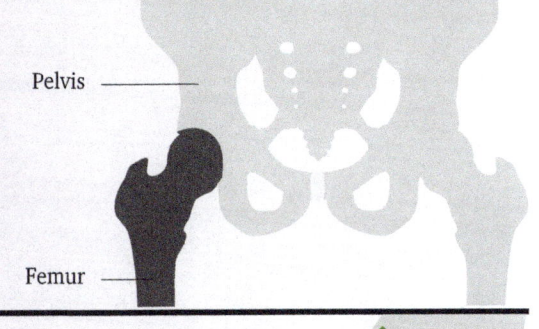 Pelvis Femur
Hip Extensors	Muscles at the back of the legs that extend the legs to the back. They include: Glutes Hamstrings Adductor Magnus	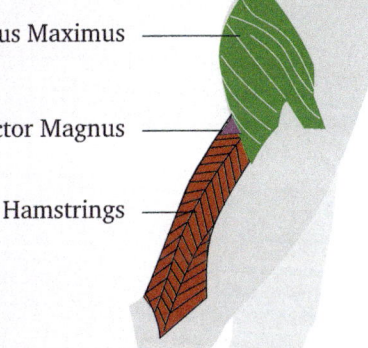 Gluteus Maximus Adductor Magnus Hamstrings

FUNDAMENTALS 147

Hip Flexors	Muscles at the front of the hip that lift the thigh toward the torso. The main muscle of the Hip Flexors is the Psoas.	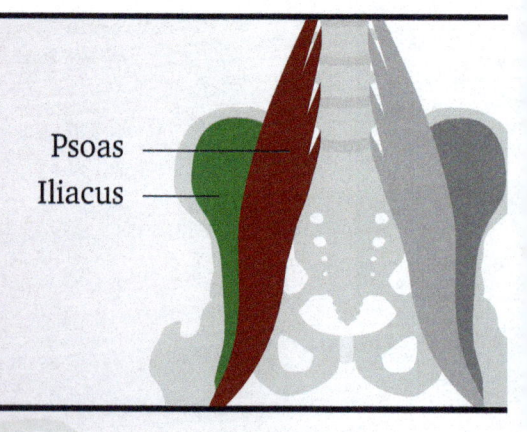 Psoas, Iliacus
Intercostal Muscles	The muscles between the ribs that help to expand and contract the space between each rib. These muscles aid in breathing.	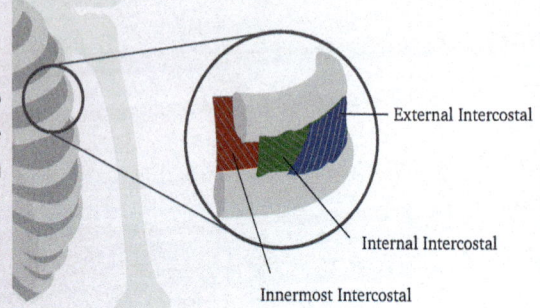 External Intercostal, Internal Intercostal, Innermost Intercostal
Internal Abdominal Obliques	The muscles at the side of the abdominals that twist or rotate the spine. Internal Abdominal Obliques help to stabilize the hips. Working together, the larger External Abdominal Obliques covers the Internal Abdominal Obliques.	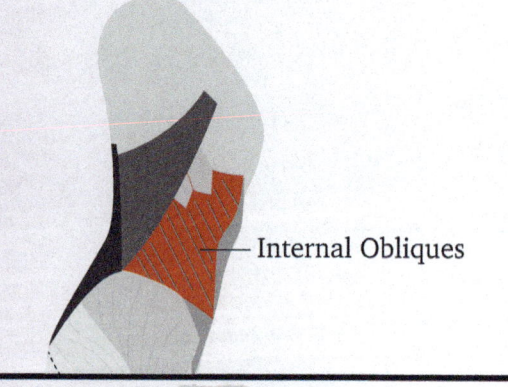 Internal Obliques
Latissimus Dorsi	The biggest muscle in the back and assists in extending the spine. (Back-bending).	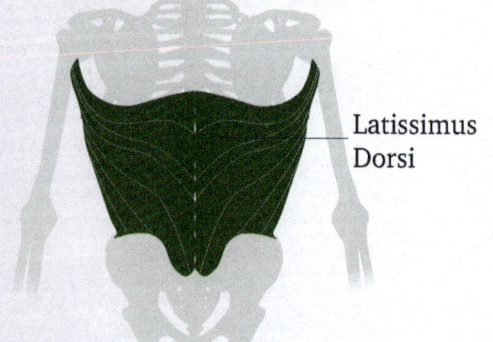 Latissimus Dorsi

Levator Scapulae

Levator Scapulae is situated at the back and side of the neck. Its main function is the elevate the Scapula (Shoulder blade).

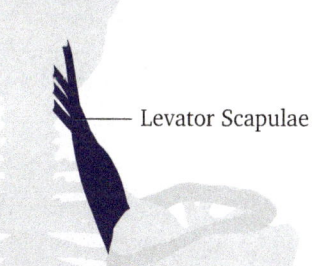

Lumbar Spine

Lumbar spine is located in the lower back and consists of 5 Vertebrae between the bottom ribs and pelvis. L1 to L5. The Lumbar spine helps support the weight of the upper torso and includes the head and neck. The lumbar spine also transfers weight from the upper body to the legs.

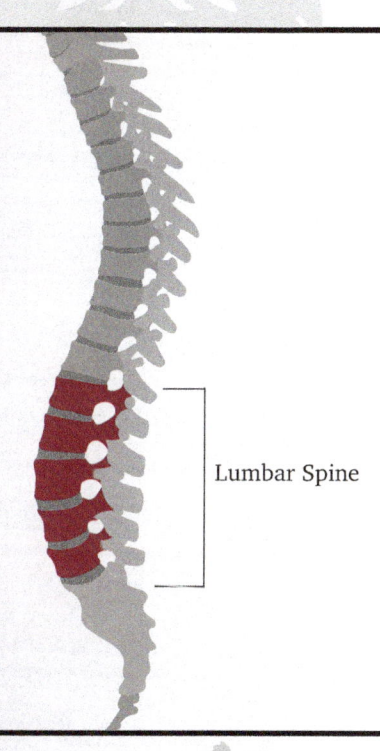

Multifidus Muscles

Multifidi muscles is the full length of muscles along the spinal column. Multifidus muscle plays an important role in stabilizing the joints within the spine. Multifidi muscles are stronger and more developed in the lumbar spine.

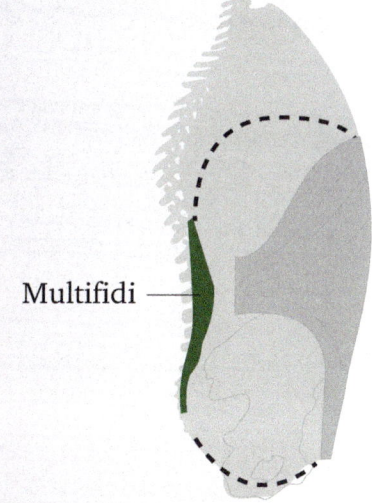

FUNDAMENTALS 149

Paraspinals

Paraspinals, also known as Erector Spinae, are located along the spine. This important muscle group supports the back during side to side bending, extension and twisting of the torso.

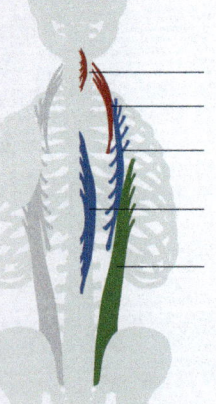

- Spinalis Cervicis
- Iliocostalis Cervicis
- Iliocostalis Thoracis
- Spinalis Thoracis
- Iliocostalis Lumborum

Pectorals

Referred to as "pecs", they live on both right and left side of the chest and consist of four muscles. The pectorals are predominantly used to control the movement of the arms.

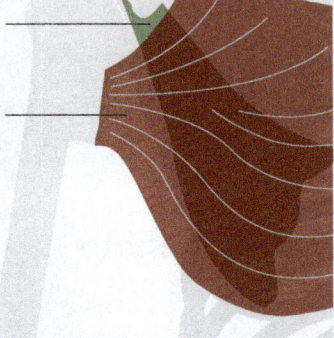

- Pectoralis Minor
- Pectoralis Major

Pelvis

A basin-shaped structure of the vertebrate skeleton, composed of the unnamed bones on the sides, the pubis in front, and the sacrum and coccyx (tailbone) behind, that rests on the lower limbs and supports the spinal column. The main function of the pelvis is to support the upper body and transfer body weight to the lower limbs. The pelvis also serves as the site of attachment for multiple muscles.

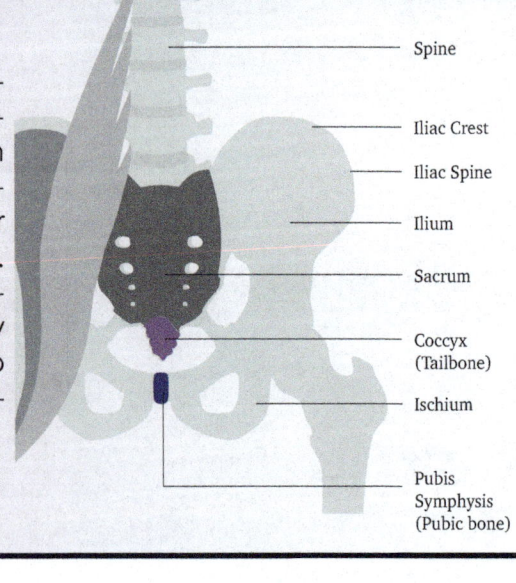

- Spine
- Iliac Crest
- Iliac Spine
- Ilium
- Sacrum
- Coccyx (Tailbone)
- Ischium
- Pubis Symphysis (Pubic bone)

Quadratus Lumborum

Referred to as "QL". This is the deepest of muscle in the lower back. It is found in the lower back between the lower ribs and the pelvis. The QL aids in breathing, side to side motion and back-bending.

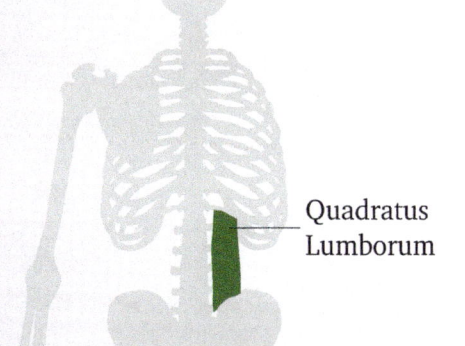

Quadratus Lumborum

Quadriceps

Muscles of the front of the thigh, from the hip to the knee, that makes up the major muscles of the thigh. The quadriceps work to straighten the knee, flexes the hip, adduct the thigh and also extends and externally rotates the thigh and stabilizes the kneecap.

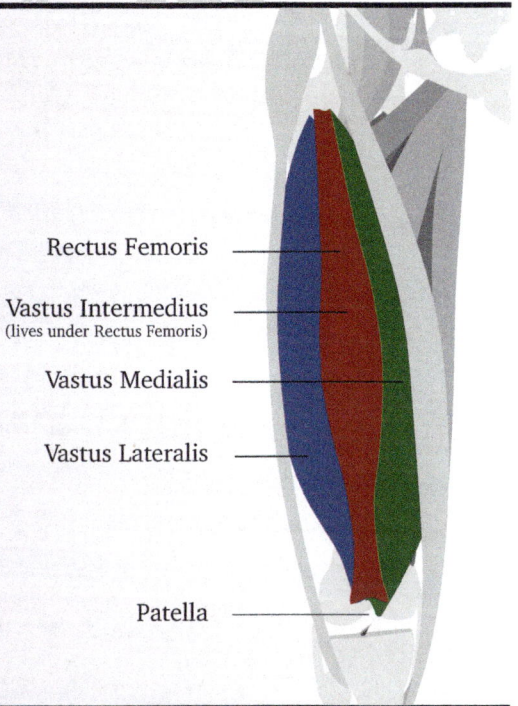

Rectus Femoris

Vastus Intermedius
(lives under Rectus Femoris)

Vastus Medialis

Vastus Lateralis

Patella

Rectus Abdominus

The muscles in the front of the abdomen, also known as the "six pack", that run from the bottom of the sternum to the pubic bone and assists in flexing the spine.

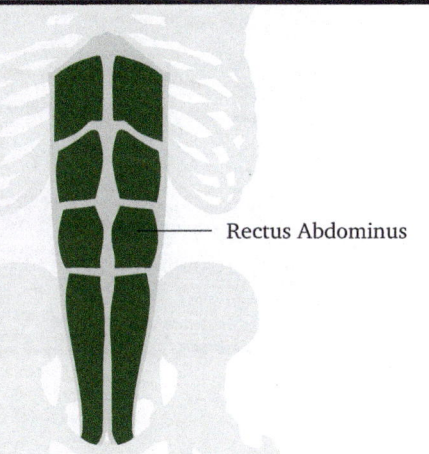

Rectus Abdominus

FUNDAMENTALS

Rhomboids

Muscles located at the upper thoracic spine, that retracts and elevate the scapula (the inner border of shoulder blade)

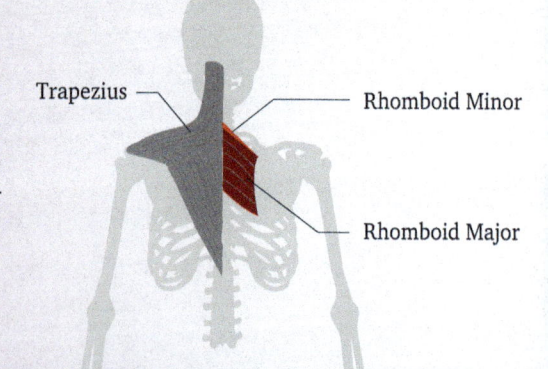

Scapular Stabilizers

A group of 5 muscles that are used to elevate (lifting shoulders to ears), depress (slide the shoulders down the back) and retract (bringing the shoulder blades together).

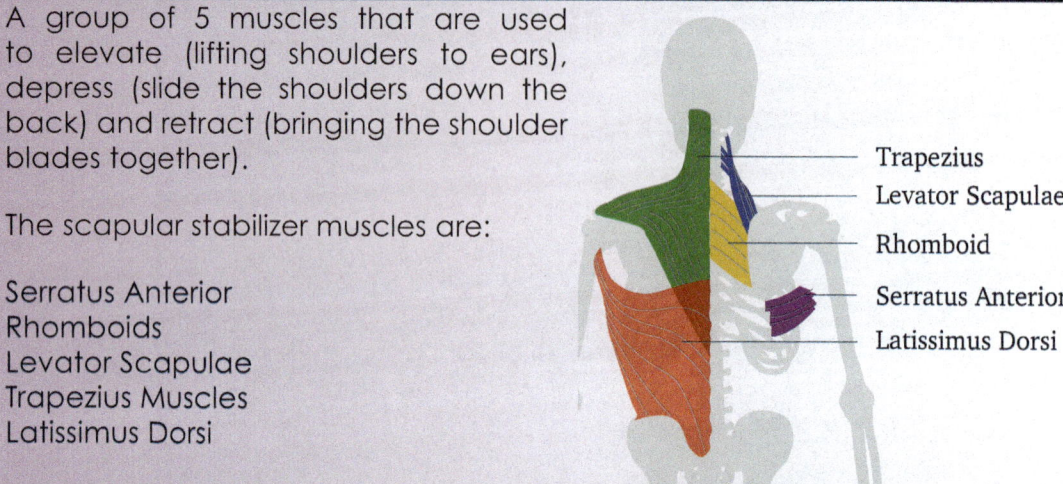

The scapular stabilizer muscles are:

Serratus Anterior
Rhomboids
Levator Scapulae
Trapezius Muscles
Latissimus Dorsi

Serratus Anterior

Serratus Anterior is a fan-shaped muscle that spreads across the upper 8 or 9 Vertebrae. This muscle helps to move the shoulder blade forward and up.

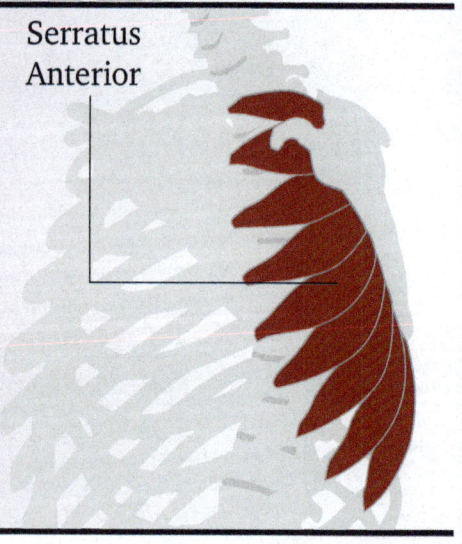

Serratus Posterior

Serratus Posterior extends diagonally from the vertebral column to the rib cage. This muscle draws the rips downward and backward and assists in twisting and extending the torso. It also contributes to inhalation and forced exhalation of air from the lungs.

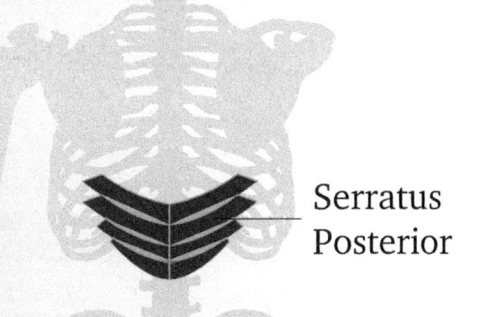

— Serratus Posterior

Sitting Bones

Sitting Bones, also called Sits Bones or Sitz Bones, are located at the bottom of the Pelvis. The anatomical name is Ischial Tuberosity. When you sit upright, you are balancing on your Sitting Bones.

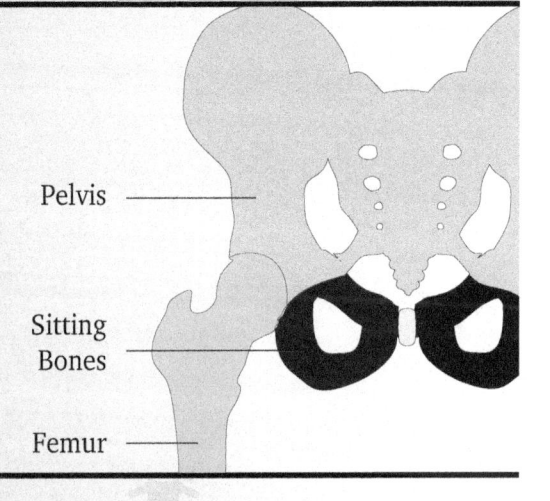

Pelvis

Sitting Bones

Femur

Sternum

The sternum is the flat breast bone at the front of the chest. It connects to the ribs via cartilage and forms the front of the rib cage. The sternum aids in opening up the front of the chest.

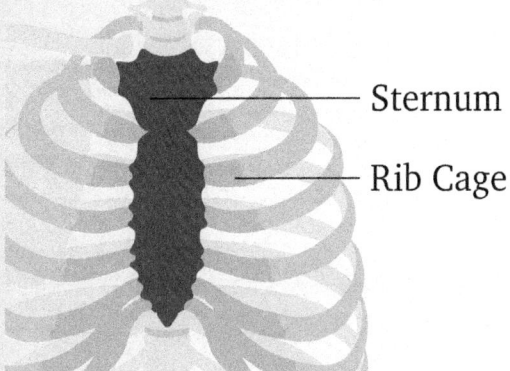

Sternum

Rib Cage

FUNDAMENTALS

Teres Major and Teres Minor

Teres Minor: Just below the shoulder joint and draws the arm toward the torso and rotates the arm upwards.

Teres Major: Also just below the shoulder joint and assists in rotating the arm outward.

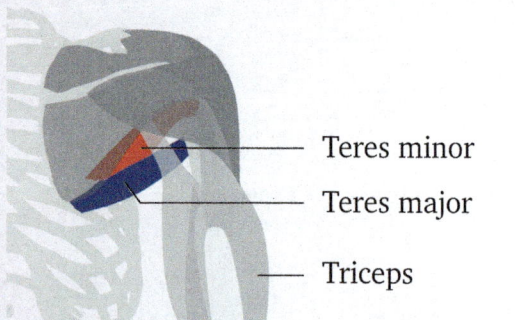

- Teres minor
- Teres major
- Triceps

Thoracic Spine

The thoracic spine is comprised of twelve vertebral bodies (T1-T12) that make up the mid-region of the spine. This section of the spine has a kyphotic curve (C-shape). The firm attachment to the rib cage at each level of the thoracic spine provides stability and structural support and allows very little articulation.

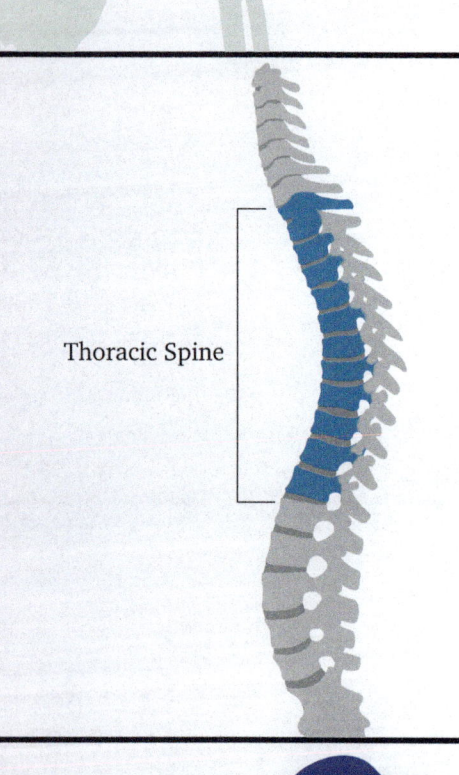

Thoracic Spine

Torso

The torso is an anatomical term for the central part, or core, from where the neck and limbs extend.

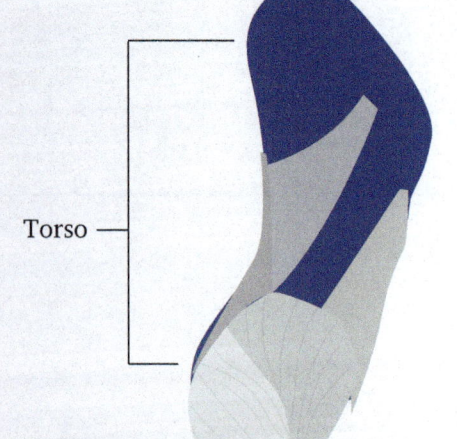

Torso

154 EXTRAS

Transverse Abdominus

Transverse Abdominus is one of the four muscles of the Abdominals and is located front and side of the deep abdominal wall. It is an important muscle that acts as a stabilizer for the back and core muscles.

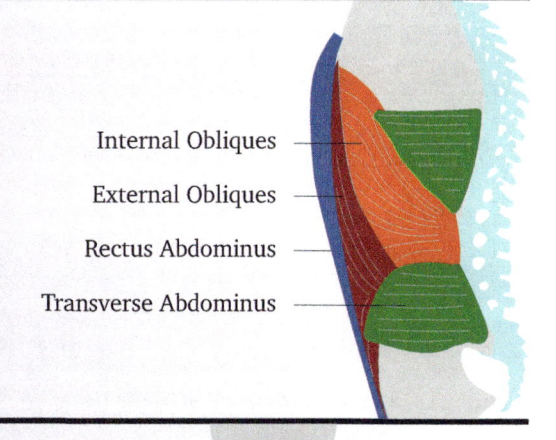

- Internal Obliques
- External Obliques
- Rectus Abdominus
- Transverse Abdominus

Trapezius: Upper, Middle and Lower

Muscle group that extends from the occipital bone (skull-bone) down to the lower thoracic spine and laterally to the spine of the scapula. They move the scapulae and support the arms.

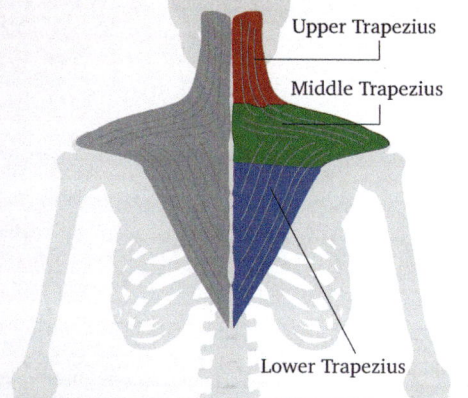

- Upper Trapezius
- Middle Trapezius
- Lower Trapezius

Triceps

The large muscle on the back of the upper arm. The triceps are one of the muscles that assists in straightening the elbow joint.

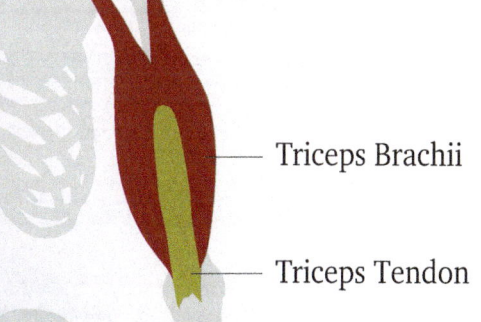

- Triceps Brachii
- Triceps Tendon

FUNDAMENTALS

Vertebrae

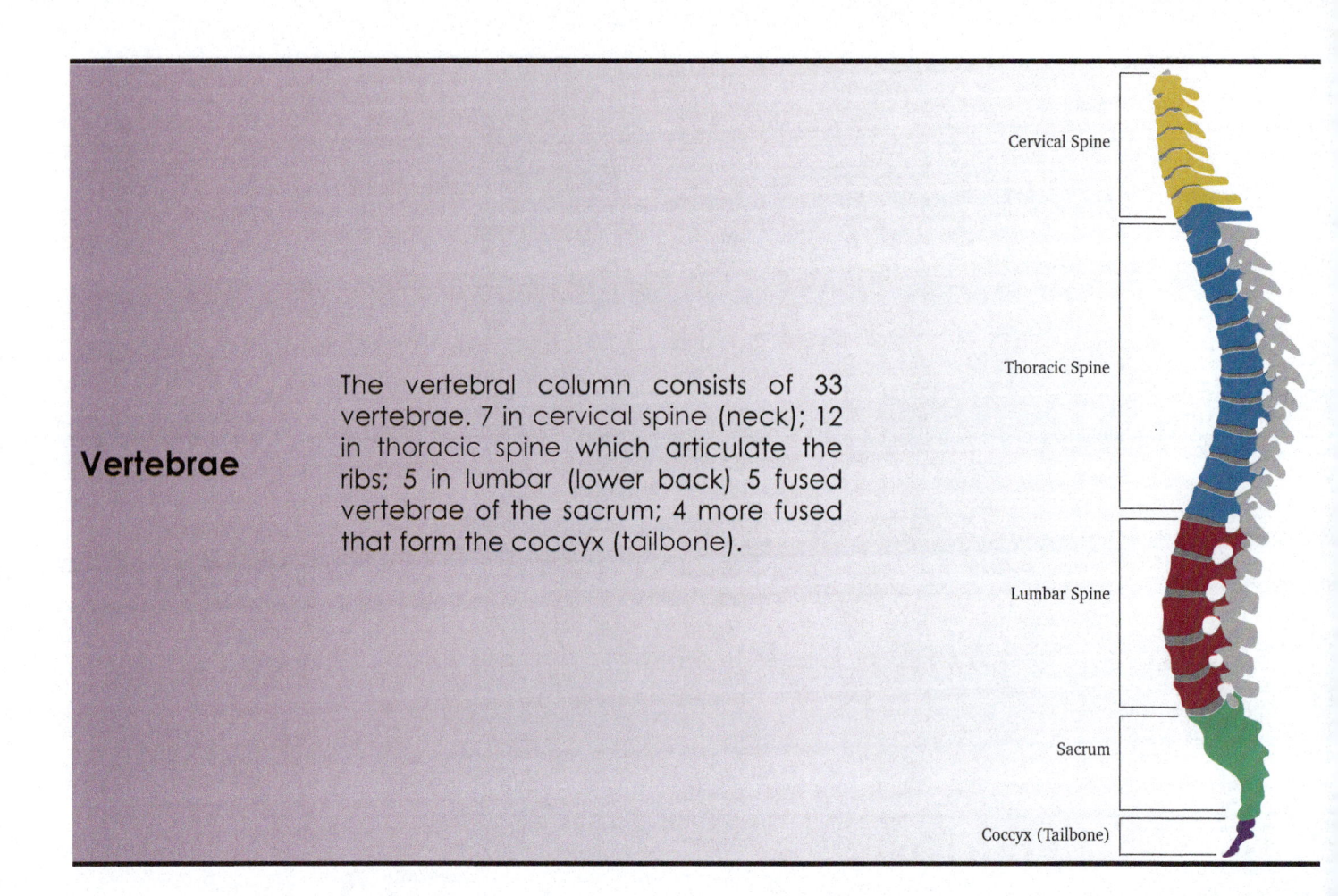

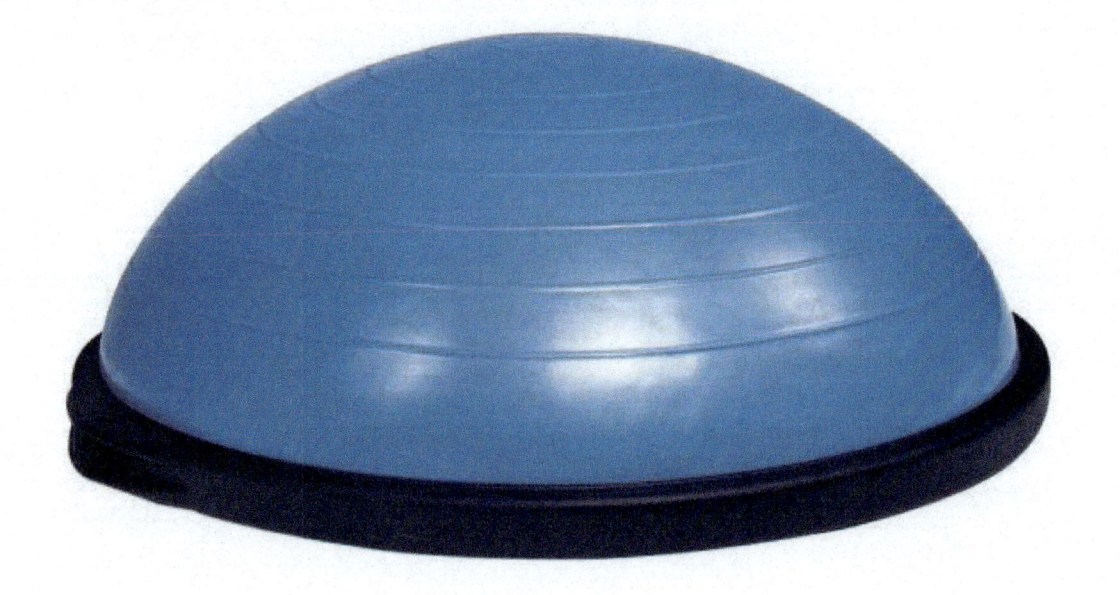

The vertebral column consists of 33 vertebrae. 7 in cervical spine (neck); 12 in thoracic spine which articulate the ribs; 5 in lumbar (lower back) 5 fused vertebrae of the sacrum; 4 more fused that form the coccyx (tailbone).

Cervical Spine

Thoracic Spine

Lumbar Spine

Sacrum

Coccyx (Tailbone)

FUNDAMENTAL MINI WORKOUTS

ABDOMINALS

1. Spinal Mobilization (Exercise 1) .... page 18

2. Tip Upper Body Side to Side (Exercise 5) .... page 28

3. Child's Pose (Exercise 10) .... page 38

4. Hundred (Exercise 11) .... page 40

5. Half Roll Back (Exercise 12) .... page 43

6. Roll Up Prep (Exercise 13) .... page 45

7. Single Leg Circle (Exercise 14) .... page 48

8. Sitting Spine Twist (Exercise 15) .... page 50

9. Single Leg Stretch Prep (Exercise 17) .... page 55

10. Child's Pose (Exercise 10) .... page 38

FUNDAMENTALS

GLUTES AND LEGS (Do Full Exercises-Unless Noted)

11. Spinal Mobilization (Exercise 1-Lower Spine Mobilization) .... page 18

12. Shoulder Bridge Prep (Exercise 20) .... page 64

13. Single Leg Stretch Prep (Exercise 17) .... page 55

14. Double Leg Stretch Prep (Exercise 18) .... page 59

15. Roll Over Prep (Exercise 21) .... page 68

16. Double Leg Extension Prep (Exercise 22) .... page 70

17. Single Leg Kick (Exercise 23) .... page 73

18. Saw (Exercise 24) .... page 75

19. Sitting Spine Stretch Forward (Exercise 31) .... page 102

20. Swimming Prep (Exercise 33) .... page 107

21. Side Leg Lift Series (Exercise 29) .... page 95

22. Side Lying Clam Series (Exercise 28 - Sub Exercise 1) .... page 87

23. Mermaid (Exercise 45) .... page 141

ABS AND ARMS (Do Full Exercises-Unless Noted)

1. Abdominals (Exercise 8) .... page 34

2. Hundred (Exercise 11) .... page 40

3. Teaser Prep (Exercise 27) .... page 84

4. Scissors Prep (Exercise 19) .... page 61

5. Side Leg Lift Series (Exercise 29 -Sub-Exercise 2) .... page 97

6. Leg Pull Front Prep (Exercise 34) .... page 110

7. Reverse Plank Prep (Leg Pull) (Exercise 35) .... page 112

8. Neck Pull Prep (Exercise 25) .... page 78

9. Pilates Push-Up Prep 1 (Exercise 36) .... page 115

10. Elbow Plank Prep (Exercise 37) .... page 118

11. Side Bend Prep (Exercise 40) .... page 124

12. Cat Stretch (Exercise 30) .... page 99

13. Shoulder Bridge Prep (Exercise 20) .... page 64

14. Seal (Exercise 44) .... page 139

FUNDAMENTALS 159

FULL BODY CHALLENGE (Do Following Modifications)

1. **Abdominals (Exercise 8)**

   - **Modification #2:** Head, shoulders and spine on mat, legs over the top of dome.. page 35

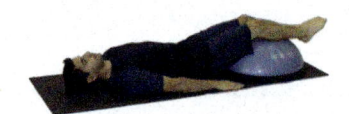

2. **Breast Stroke Prep (Exercise 9)**

   - **Modification #2:** Torpedo prep. Straighten the knees, feet are flexed on the mat ....page 37

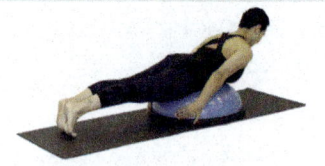

3. **Swan Dive Prep (Exercise 32)**

   - **Modification #2:** Lift and lower the legs only........................page 106

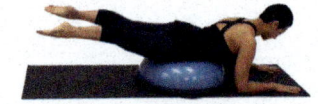

4. **Child's Pose (Exercise 10)**

   - **Modification #3:** Shins on the dome. Knees and ankles together. Push hands into the mat .... page 39

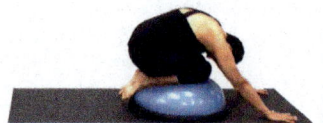

5. **Side Leg Lift Series (Exercise 29)**

   - **Sub Exercise 1, Modification #2:** Keep the top foot flexed and tap in front and behind the bottom leg ....page 96

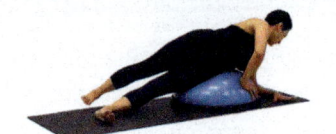

   - **Sub Exercise 2, Modification #1:** Circle the leg with flexed foot. Hand on the hip or on the dome.. ....page 97

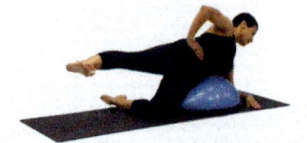

6. **Side Bend Prep (Exercise 40)**

   - **Modification #3:** On elbow with hips up, straighten and bend the bottom leg only..page 126

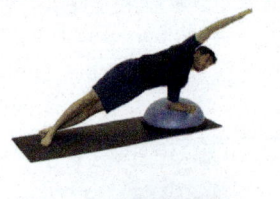

   - **Modification #6:** L elbow on mat, L knee on mat and extend the L leg behind the R leg. ....page 127

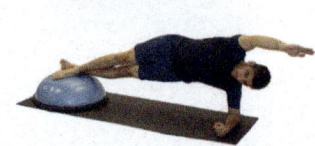

7. **Hundred (Exercise 11)**

   • **Modification #3:** Flat side up. Curl forward and place one hand behind the head. .... page 41

8. **Seal (Exercise 44)**

   • **Modification #2:** Feet clap 3 times for balance and control. Sit further away from the dome. ....page 140

9. **Roll Up Prep (Exercise 13)**

   • **Modification #2:** Legs can stay bent throughout the roll-ups. .... page 46

10. **Double Leg Extension Prep (Exercise 22)**

    • **Modification #2:** Circle extended leg .... page 71

    • **Modification #3:** Pulse extended legs upwards. Legs apart or together. ....page 71

    • **Modification #5:** Legs hovering flex and point both feet in extension...page 71

11. **Single Leg Stretch Prep (Exercise 17)**

    • **Modification #1:** Hands behind the head. Slide one leg out hovering above the mat. Alternate sides ....page 57

12. **Double Leg Stretch Prep (Exercise 18)**

    • **Modification #1:** Hands behind the head – from straight legs to bent knees...page 60

    • **Modification #2:** Double knee lift..page 60

FUNDAMENTALS   161

13. **Obliques Roll Back (Exercise 26)**

- **Modification #2:** Knees and feet together
  or slightly apart. ....page 82

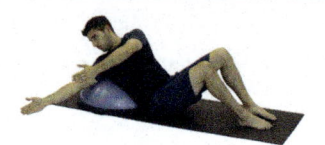

14. **Sitting Spine Stretch Forward (Exercise 31)**

- **Modification #1:** Straight legs wider
  than hip distance apart ....page 103

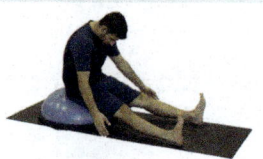

- **Modification #2:** Flat side up. Keep the dome level as you curl
  forward and back up ....page 103

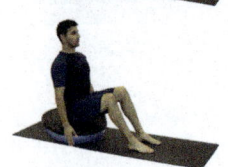

15. **Swimming Prep (Exercise 33)**

- **Modification #2:** Lift both arms together with knees bent
  or straight legs. ....page 108

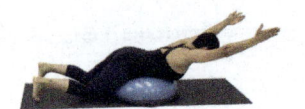

- **Modification #3:** Lift both legs together,
  elbows slightly bent ....page 108

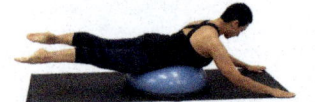

- **Modification #4:** Flat side up. Keep hands on mat,
  lift legs only ....page 109

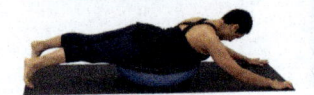

16. **Mermaid (Exercise 45)**

- **Modification #1:** Support head with bottom hand
  and lean back. ....page 142

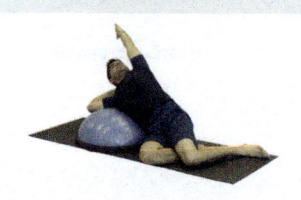

RESOURCES

BOOKS

Get On It!: BOSU® Balance Trainer
   Author: Miriane Taylor, Jane Aronovitch, Colleen Craig
   Publisher: Ulysses Press
   ISBN-10: 1-56975-589-2
   ISBN-13: 978-1-56975-589-1
   Book Search www.amazon.com for: Get On It!: BOSU

Pilates on the Ball
   Author: Colleen Craig
   Publisher: Healing Arts Press
   ISBN: 089281981-2
   Book Search www.amazon.com for: Pilates on the Ball

Abs on the Ball
   Author: Colleen Craig
   Publisher: Healing Arts Press
   ISBN: 089281098
   Book Search www.amazon.com for: Abs on the Ball

Strength Training on the Ball
   Author: Colleen Craig
   Publisher: Healing Arts Press
   ISBN: 159477011-5
   Book Search www.amazon.com for: Strength Training on the Ball

The Pilates Powerhouse
   Author: Mari Winsor
   Publisher: Perseus Books
   ISBN: 0-7382-0228-2
   Book Search www.amazon.com for: The Pilates Powerhouse

Pilates' Return to Life Through Contrology
   Author: Joseph Pilates, Judd Robbins
   Publisher: Presentation Dynamics
   ISBN-10: 1928564909
   ISBN-13: 978-1928564904
   Book Search www.amazon.com for: Pilates' Return to Life Through Contrology

The Great Balance and Stability Handbook
   Author: Andre Noel Potvin and Chad Benson
   Publisher: Productive Fitness Products Inc.
   ISBN: 0-9731262-0-5
   Book Search www.amazon.com for: The Great Balance and Stability Handbook

FUNDAMENTALS

Pilates Anatomy
    Author: Dr. Abigail Ellsworth
    Publisher: Thunder Bay Press
    ISBN-10: 978-1-60710-015-7
    ISBN-13: 1-60710-015-0
    Book Search www.amazon.com for: Pilates Anatomy Ellsworth

Integrated Balance Training *(A Programming Guide for Fitness and Health Professionals)*
    Author: Douglas Brooks M.S.
    Publisher: DW Fitness, LLC (January 1, 2002)
    ISBN-10 : 1878655094
    ISBN-13 : 978-1878655097
    Book Search www.amazon.com for: Integrated Balance Training

VIDEOS

- **Pilates on the Ball DVD:** http://pilatesontheball.com
- **BOSU Team Videos:** www.bosu.com/videos
- **Winsor Pilates:** https://winsorpilates.intelivideo.com/discovery

WEBSITES

- **Taylor'd Pilates:** www.taylor-dpilates.com
- **Pilates on the Ball:** www.pilatesontheball.com
- **David Weck BOSU Team:** www.bosu.com
- **Where to Purchase BOSU** https://www.bosu.com/bosu-pro-balance-trainers
- **PHD Software** www.phdsoftware.com
- **Sana Khan Photography** Sana Khan Photography
- **Daub and Design** www.daubanddesign.com

PILATES ON THE BOSU® TEAM

We don't do average, we do **AWESOME**.

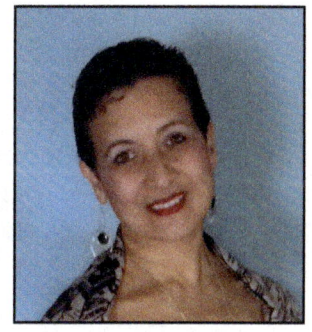

MIRIANE TAYLOR (Author/Model/Team Leader)
A book is only as good as its team and I warmly acknowledge the contribution of the following team members in bringing this book to life:

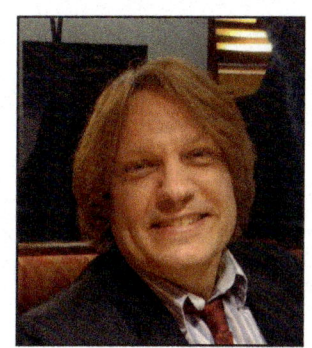

EDDIE KASTRAU (Copy Editor/Layout/Photographer)
Eddie's amazing technical computer skills has made "Pilates on the BOSU" an eye-catching sensation. Having studied robotics and industrial electricity before pursuing a dance career, culminating as a performer with the Danny Grossman Dance Company for 30 years. At present, Eddie is actively teaching the Grossman dance repertoire as well as being the archival preservationist for numerous dance companies. His artistic sensibility is perfectly balanced with his logical mind.

I had the pleasure of dancing with Eddie in my early years as a contemporary dancer in Toronto. Thank you for making every moment working with you such a breathtaking experience, solving all the dilemmas and issues with such ease and grace. I adore your energy, your infinite well of patience and your diligence. Thank you for making "Pilates on the BOSU" a reality. I look forward to creating many more magical projects with you.

COLLEEN CRAIG *(Forward Contributor)*
Colleen is a certified Pilates instructor and author of 3 books about Pilates on the exercise ball.

I met Colleen at Stott Pilates studio in Toronto, where I received my teacher training in Pilates. I am eternally grateful for all you have done to encourage me to complete "Pilates on the BOSU". Thank you for taking the time to give me feedback and tips. Sharing your knowledge and your expertise is and always will be priceless. "Pilates on the BOSU" is greatly enriched because of your guidance.

NADIM HABIB (Model)
Nadim studied Business Tourism and Environmental Science, Finance and Day Trading, all the while educating himself on Nutrition. Nadim began his Pilates work with Miriane in 2014 and has continued a daily workout regime that includes the BOSU. "The BOSU is such an integral part of my life, my strength and my fluidity of movement."

My protégé, my star student of Pilates. Thank you for your pure kind heart and generous soul. Always there no matter what. Thank you for showing me the side of mankind that continues to glow. For taking time out of your schedule while taking such good care of your mom. I really appreciate your friendship and am forever grateful and blessed to know you.

FUNDAMENTALS

CHARMAINE HEW WING (Graphic Artist)
Charmaine is currently working for a large Toronto firm as supervisor of multimedia and publishing, creating graphic designs for presentations and marketing materials. Charmaine believes in pursuing your dreams and that one is only limited by what they believe. Though it's taken her 30 years, she is currently completing her undergraduate pre-med degree, while working full-time, in order to realize her lifelong dream of becoming a doctor. Combining these two passions, Charmaine created wonderful anatomical illustrations for this book.

Charmaine you have been on this Journey of writing "Pilates on the BOSU" since 2006. Doing Pilates with me while simultaneously preparing workout charts, manuals and handouts to students that was second to none. Thank you for sharing so much of your time to make me look amazing at all my seminars and workshops all over the world and that includes "Get on it" BOSU. Your genuine friendship and heart is very much appreciated.

SANA KHAN (Photographer)
Sana is a Technology Analyst and Freelance Photographer. Her wonderful photographic skills and her tremendous eye for detail, were put to good use in "*Pilates on the BOSU*".

What an amazing first meeting we had in our gym. Your love and gift for photography, your professional presentation, your stunning self, shines through everything that you do. Thank you for sharing your love of photography that has made the models and books come to life. This is just the beginning of many more amazing projects that awaits you. Continue to share your skills with the world.

CAROL ANDERSON (Copy Editor)
Carol is a dance artist, choreographer, writer, educator and a founding member of Dancemakers. She is the author of numerous articles on Canadian dance and dancers, since 1997 has written thirty-seven editions of "Carol's Dance Notes," and has authored, co-authored and edited twelve books.

I have admired you since the first day I saw you on stage. Spellbound! is the word I can use to describe you. When I was told that you are editing and writing I jumped at the chance to have your guidance with "Pilates on the BOSU". Thank you making editing this book so seamless. It is such an honor to know you and to work with you. My heart is forever grateful.

LEXI SOURKOREFO (Costume Designer and Builder)
Lexi artfully blends colour and texture to create unique works, using surface design techniques to make recognizable, one of a kind garments - tailored for the everyday and active lifestyle.

I feel so blessed to have been introduced to you. Your workout clothes are so comfortable and stunning to wear. Thank you for letting me include your clothing line in my book. Daub and Design is a must wear for everyone.

BRIAN TAYLOR (Photographer/Patron)
Brian's patience and attention to detail were meticulously honed while Brian was a transit driver for 29 years, making him an ideal candidate as a supporter of a book writer.

My wonderful and awesome husband with so much patience. Thank you for putting up with me. I am sure I drove you crazy during this process of writing "Pilates on the BOSU". I am grateful for your love and support. Thank you for being my rock.

GRETA GOLICK (Pilates Student/Inspirator)
Besides a Pilates student of Miriane, Dr. Greta Golick was an assistant professor at the Faculty of Information, University of Toronto. She taught foundation courses in Book History and Print Culture Collaboration.

I dedicate this book to my friend Greta Golick. Forever in my heart. Thank you for sharing and teaching so much about yourself. Thank you for sharing your love of books. Thank you for being my angel. I remember the words you shared: "You are on top of the mountain, you have come too far to stop now." I cannot tell you just how much those words have kept me going. I miss you dearly.

After you have mastered Pilates on the BOSU: Fundamentals, be sure to explore the next book, Pilates on the BOSU: Intermediate (coming soon).

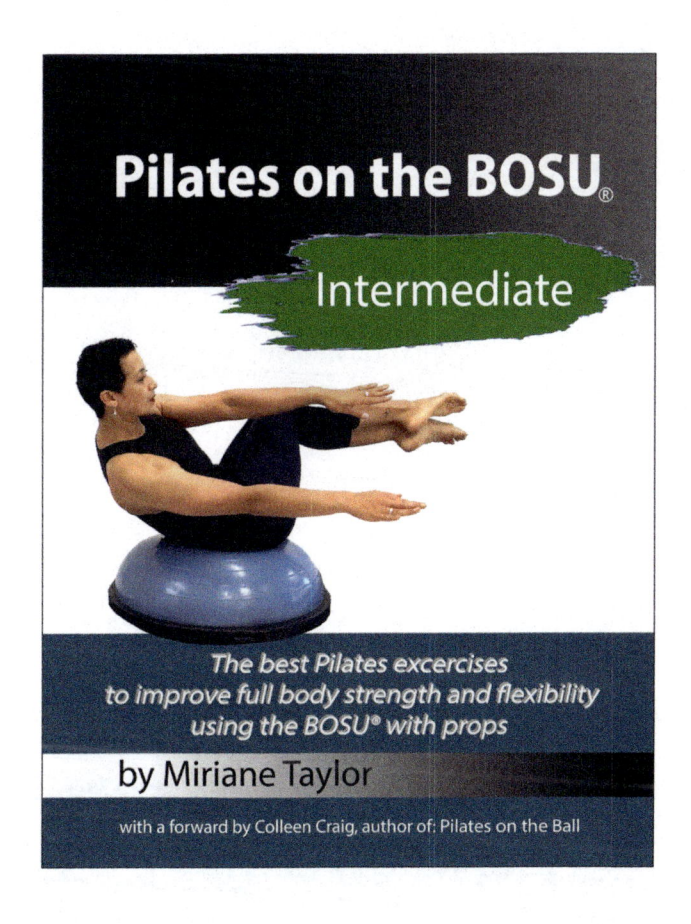

taylor d
PILATES

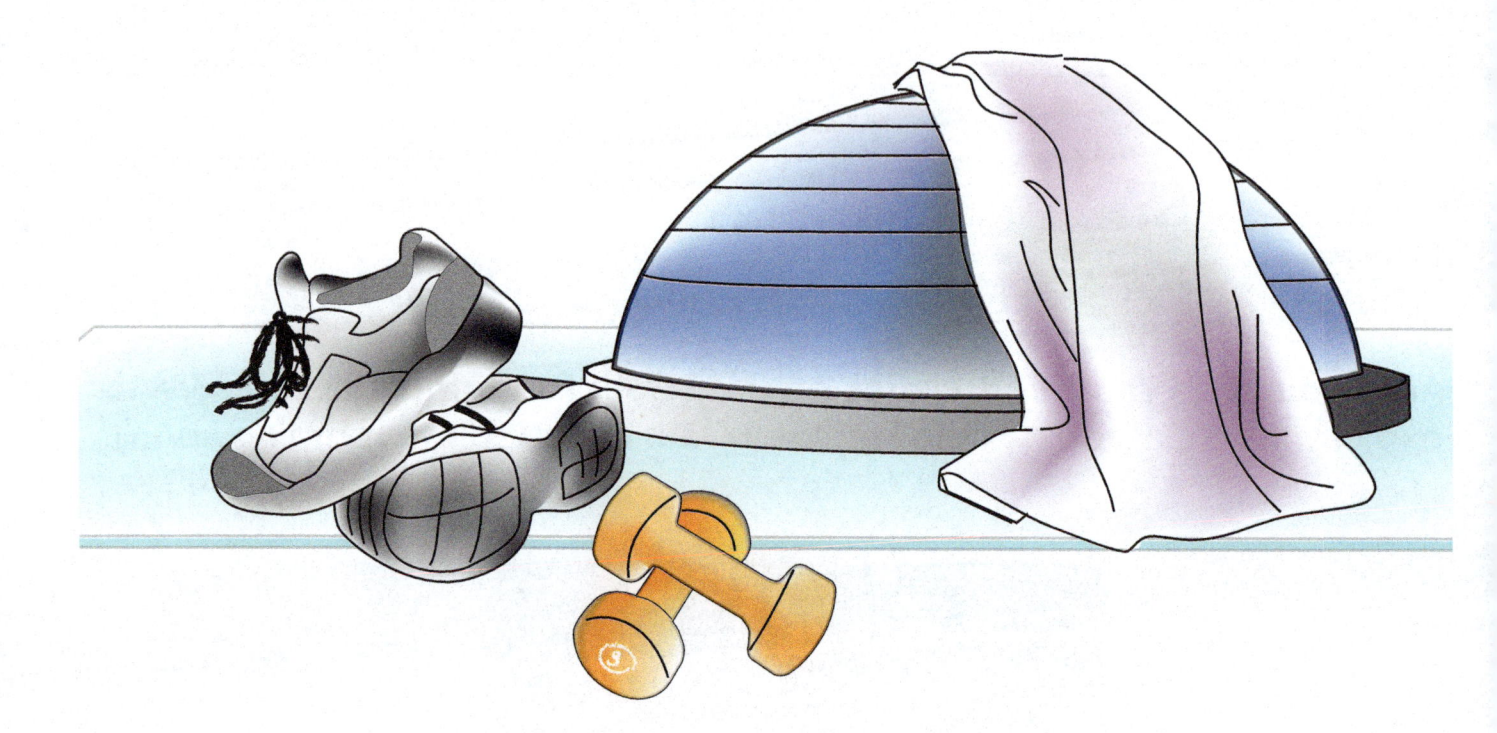

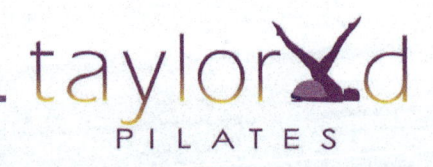

www.taylor-dpilates.com

Printed in Great Britain
by Amazon